Aaa ElDin Kassem

Maha Marzouk

Metronidazole "Controlled Release Delivery Systems"

Dalia AbdelRhman
Alaa ElDin Kassem
Maha Marzouk

Metronidazole "Controlled Release Delivery Systems"

LAP LAMBERT Academic Publishing

Imprint

Any brand names and product names mentioned in this book are subject to trademark, brand or patent protection and are trademarks or registered trademarks of their respective holders. The use of brand names, product names, common names, trade names, product descriptions etc. even without a particular marking in this work is in no way to be construed to mean that such names may be regarded as unrestricted in respect of trademark and brand protection legislation and could thus be used by anyone.

Cover image: www.ingimage.com

Publisher:
LAP LAMBERT Academic Publishing
is a trademark of
International Book Market Service Ltd., member of OmniScriptum Publishing Group
17 Meldrum Street, Beau Bassin 71504, Mauritius

ISBN: 978-3-659-53230-6

Copyright © Dalia AbdelRhman, Alaa ElDin Kassem, Maha Marzouk
Copyright © 2014 International Book Market Service Ltd., member of OmniScriptum Publishing Group

CONTENTS

ACKNOWLEDGEMENTS

I am deeply thankful to **GOD** by the grace of whom the present work was realized.

This thesis would not have been possible without the endless help, support, advice, and patience of my supervisor **Prof.Dr.ALAA EL-DIN ALi KASSEM** Professor of pharmaceutics and Dean of Faculty of pharmacy for Girls, Al- Azhar University, throughout the work. I owe you.

I am profoundly grateful to my supervisor **Dr.Maha Abdel-Hameed Marzouk**, Lecturer of pharmaceutics, Faculty of pharmacy, Al-Azhar University for constant guidance and continuous help throughout the work.

I wish to express my heartly appreciation to Prof.Dr.ABD-ALLAH EL DESOKY, Head of Production section, EIPICO Co., for his kindly assistance.

I wish to express my deepest thankfulness to the staff of EIPICO CO, 10th of Ramadan City, Egypt (particularly Dr. MAGDA IBRAHIM Manager of Control section and Analyst AHMED REFAAT) who kindly helped me during in-vivo study.

I would also like to thank the volunteers (members of physician stuff in al-Hussin hospital) who, gladly, gave up their time and blood to participate in the in-vivo study carried out during this work.

Finally, endless thanks go to my mum, dad, brother, husband, and daughters who, in their own ways, have provided love, support and understanding during my extended further education.

To my family, whose vision, enthusiasm, and answering support helped to make a lifelong dream come true.

ABSTRACT

Many pharmaceutical investigations have been carried out to develop oral controlled release drug delivery system. Controlled release (CR) implies predictability and reproducibility in the drug release kinetics, i.e., attempts to control drug concentrations in the target tissue. One of the most recent approaches to control the release of the drugs is the floating drug delivery system.

Floating drug delivery systems or hydrodynamic balanced systems have a bulk density lower than gastric fluids and thus remain buoyant in the stomach without affecting the gastric emptying rate for a prolonged period of time. While the system is floating on the gastric contents, the drug is released slowly at a desired rate from the system. After the release of drug, the residual system is emptied from the stomach. This results in an increase in the gastric residence time and a better control of fluctuations in plasma drug concentrations in some cases.

Various attempts have been made to develop floating systems to control drug release; among them is the so called hydrodynamic balanced system (HBS). Such a system is useful for drugs acting locally in the proximal gastrointestinal tract or for drugs that degraded in the intestinal fluids; metronidazole (the drug used in this thesis) is one drug from the former category.

In this work an antimicrobial drug metronidazole was introduced as model drug to control its release in the stomach through the formation of different floating system to exert its local effect in the stomach.

Accordingly, the aim of this thesis was the formulation of metronidazole as different pharmaceutical preparations (tablets, capsules and hollow microspheres) in a controlled release floating form by addition of different polymers with different ratios.

The specific work under taken in this thesis is briefly described below:

Part I: Formulation and In-vitro performance of metronidazole floating dosage forms.

Part II: Accelerated stability of metronidazole floating dosage forms.

Part III: Bioavailability of metronidazole floating dosage forms.

Part I: Formulation and In-vitro performance of metronidazole floating dosage forms.

In this part, attempts have been made to investigate special delivery system for metronidazole so as to be able for remaining buoyant on the stomach contents and increasing the stomach residence time of the drug to exert its therapeutic effect locally in the stomach for longer time. This was achieved by performing suitable floating systems.

Accordingly, this part comprises of two chapters as follow:

Chapter I: Effervescent metronidazole floating tablets

In this chapter, the current technological developments of floating drug delivery system including effervescent floating system were discussed. These buoyant delivery systems include a gas-generating component in the formulation.

The present chapter includes formulation, dissolutions, and buoyancy of sustained release tablet of metronidazole, then preparation of floating bilayer compressed tablets which is applied for formulae that gave the best result of sustained action of metronidazole (be able to deliver the drug at constant rates up to 90% of the total loading dose within 6 hours).

For comparison, immediate release reference tablets containing the same dose of metronidazole (plain tablet) but without any polymer were also formulated.

The selected polymers for the floating sustained release system were HPMC 4000, HPMC 15000, CMC, Carbopol 934, sodium alginate, pectin, methyl cellulose, and ethyl cellulose. These polymers were used separately in 2:1, 1:1, 2:3, and 1:2 drug: polymer ratios. Polymers were directly compressed with drug as tablet dosage form.

Moreover the floating behavior of all prepared dosage form formulae was clarified using the USP type I dissolution apparatus without basket.

The kinetic parameters for the in-vitro release of metronidazole were determined and were analyzed in order to explain the mechanism of drug release. Specific computer program was used for this purpose. Zero-, first- and second-order kinetics as well as, controlled diffusion model, Hixson-Crowel cube root law, and Baker and Lonsdale equation were tried.

In this chapter, thirty seven floating systems for metronidazole in the form of bilayerd tablets were obtained and they were subjected to the in-vitro tests. The in-vitro performance of the prepared formulae was carried out by testing the dissolution, floating time and floating properties. For comparison reason, the in-vitro performance of plain metronidazole dosage forms was carried out.

Further more, the prepared metronidazole tablet dosage forms were evaluated for their uniformity of weight, thickness, hardness, friability, disintegration time and drug content uniformity.

The results of this chapter revealed that:

1- All the prepared metronidazole tablet formulae complied with the pharmacopoeia requirements for uniformity of weight, thickness, drug content and disintegration time, meanwhile have reasonable hardness and friability values.

2-In-vitro release of metronidazole from directly compressed tablets using different polymers in drug: polymer ratio 2:1was carried out in a medium composed of 0.1 N HCl pH 1.2 for 6 hours. The minimum release was 73% for formula 1tA (metronidazole tablets containing HPMC 15000) after 6 hours, While the maximum release of metronidazole after 6 hours was 93.1% belonging to formula 7tA (metronidazole tablet containing methyl cellulose).

3- In-vitro release of metronidazole from directly compressed tablets using different polymers in drug: polymer ratio 1:1was carried out in 0.1 N HCl pH 1.2 for 6 hours. The minimum in-vitro release of metronidazole after 6 hours was 66.5% for formula 1tB (tablets containing HPMC 15000), while the maximum release of metronidazole after 6 hours was 99.5% concerning formula 5tB (metronidazole tablet containing CMC).

4- In-vitro release of metronidazole from directly compressed tablets using different polymers in drug: polymer ratio 2:3was carried out in 0.1 N HCl pH 1.2 for 6 hours. The minimum in-vitro release of metronidazole after 6 hours was 64.2% belonged to formula 1tC (metronidazole tablets containing HPMC 15000), while the maximum release of metronidazole after 6 hours was 100% concerning formula 5tC (metronidazole tablet containing CMC).

5-In-vitro release of metronidazole from directly compressed tablets using different polymers in drug: polymer ratio 1:2 was carried out in 0.1 N HCl pH 1.2 for 6 hours. The minimum in-vitro release of metronidazole after 6 hours was 59.2% for formula 1tD (metronidazole tablets containing HPMC 15000), while the maximum release of metronidazole after 6 hours was 91.7% concerning formula 2tD (metronidazole tablet containing HPMC 4000).

6-In addition, the plain metronidazole tablets showed very rapid release of drug.

7-Regarding the floating behavior, it was found that all prepared tablet formulae which utilize the effervescent technology of floating device (CO_2 generation) showed floating time of more than 6 hours. The HPMC 4000 content used together with the presence of gas generating mixture ($NaHCO_3$, $CaCo_3$) were satisfactory enough to keep the formula floating all the needed time.

8- The in-vitro release of metronidazole from the investigated tablet dosage forms followed different kinetic orders and no one kinetic order can explain the drug release from the specific polymer.

Chapter II: Non- Effervescent metronidazole floating preparations

This chapter investigate development of non effervescent floating preparations of locally acting metronidazole including preparation of single-unit systems (floating capsules), and multiple-unit systems (floating hollow microspheres or microballoons).The in-vitro release of metronidazole from the different preparations prepared with different ratios of various polymers as well as the various approaches used in and their mechanism of buoyancy are discussed in the following chapter.

For comparison, immediate release reference capsules and microspheres containing the same dose of metronidazole without polymer were also formulated.

The selected polymers for the floating sustained release capsules were HPMC 4000, HPMC 15000, CMC, Carbopol 934, sodium alginate, pectin, methyl cellulose, and ethyl cellulose. These polymers were used separately in 2:1, 1:1, 2:3, and 1:2 drug: polymer ratios. Formulae were simply filled to hard gelatin capsules size 00.

The floating microspheres were prepared by a modified emulsion-solvent diffusion and evaporation method using Eudragit S100 polymer in alcohol/dichloromethane mixture in drug: polymer ratio 2:1, 1:1and 1:2. The device prepared with the present technique is a polymeric microsphere with a round cavity. This microspheres was termed

12

(microballoon) due to its characteristic internal hollow structure and excellent in-vitro floatability. Metronidazole was loaded in the outer shell of the microballoon.

The prepared capsules were evaluated for their uniformity of drug content. As well as the microspheres prepared were physically evaluated for their particle size and morphology. The kinetic parameters for the in-vitro release of metronidazole were determined and analyzed in order to explain the mechanism of drug release. Specific computer program was used for this purpose.

<u>The results of this chapter revealed that:</u>

1-All the prepared metronidazole capsule formulae complied with the pharmacopoeia requirements for uniformity of drug contents.

2-In-vitro release of metronidazole from hard gelatin capsule formulae using different polymers in drug: polymer ratio 2:1was carried out in 0.1 N HCl pH 1.2 for 6 hours. The minimum release of metronidazole after 6 hours was 97.4% for formula 5cA (metronidazole capsules containing CMC).

3- In-vitro release of metronidazole from hard gelatin capsule formulae using different polymers in drug: polymer ratio 1:1was carried out in 0.1 N HCl pH 1.2 for 6 hours. The minimum in-vitro release of metronidazole after 6 hours was 87.2% concerning formula 4cB (metronidazole capsules containing sodium alginate).

4- In-vitro release of metronidazole from hard gelatin capsule formulae using different polymers in drug: polymer ratio 2:3 was carried out in 0.1

13

N HCl pH 1.2 for 6 hours. The minimum in-vitro release of metronidazole after 6 hours was 93.7% concerning formula 1cC (metronidazole capsules containing HPMC 15000).

5- In-vitro release of metronidazole from hard gelatin capsule formulae using different polymers in drug: polymer ratio 1:2 was carried out in 0.1 N HCl pH 1.2 for 6 hours. The minimum in-vitro release of metronidazole after 6 hours was 79.5% concerning formula 2cD (metronidazole capsules containing HPMC 4000).

6- Concerning the prepared formulae in capsule dosage forms which utilize non-effervescent technology of floating device, it was found that capsules containing pectin in ratio 1:2, capsules containing hydroxyl propyl methyl cellulose 15000 in both ratio 1:2, 2:3 and capsules containing hydroxyl propyl methyl cellulose 4000 in ratio 1:2 success to float over the dissolution medium for 6 hours and their % release of drug after 6 hours were 100, 86.6, 93.7, and 79.5, respectively.

7-The microspheres size of metronidazole was increased by increasing the polymer content.

8-Floating microspheres of metronidazole showed low loading efficiency due to high solubility of metronidazole in water and alcohol and its low solubility in dichloromethane, which warrants the highest escaping tendency.

9-The in-vitro release of drug was greatly retarded in case of the floating microspheres than of the plain drug or other prepared dosage forms.

14

10-Increasing the polymer content in the microspheres from drug: polymer ratio of 2:1 to 1:1 and finally 1:2 decreases the release rate of the drug.

11-Also, all the prepared formulae of microspheres showed excellent floating behaviors as all of them able to be buoyant over the dissolution medium for more than 6 hours.

12-Scanning electron microscope showed the hollow structure of all the prepared microspheres formulae with smooth surface morphology which is responsible for the buoyancy behavior of the formulae.

13-The in-vitro release of metronidazole from the investigated capsules and microspheres followed different kinetic orders and no one kinetic order can explain the drug release from the specific polymer.

Part II: Accelerated stability of metronidazole floating dosage forms.

In this part, the accelerated stability testing at 35°C and 45°C for 6 months was carried out on the selected metronidazole formulae. By applying some form of Arrhenius equation and substituting the experimentally established specific rate constants at the two elevated temperatures used, the energy of activation (Ea) and the decomposition reaction rate constant at room temperature (k_{20}) was determined. Also, t $_{1/2}$ and t $_{90}$ for each tested formulae were estimated .

A special computer program was used to determine the kinetic parameters of stability for the investigated selected metronidazole dosage form. Zero-, first- and second-order kinetics were tried to choose the most suitable order for stability study.

The obtained data showed that:

1-According to the percent of drug retained in the investigated metronidazole tablet formulae when stored at 35° C and 45°C for 6 months, it was found that the formula containing HPMC 4000 in drug: polymer ratio 2:3 showed the most stable one, while formula containing methyl cellulose in drug: polymer ratio 2:1 was the most stable one in the tested two elevated temperatures, respectively.

2-Regarding to metronidazole capsule formulae stored at 35°C and 45°C for 6 months, it was clear that the formula containing HPMC 15000 in drug: polymer ratio 2:3 showed the most stable one.

3-It was found that formula $1t_9A$ (tablet containing HPMC 15000 in drug: polymer ratio 2:1) has the highest t_{90} at 20°C according to the accelerated stability testing (2357days), while formula 7tA (tablet containing methyl cellulose in drug: polymer ratio 2:1) has the shortest t_{90} (107 days).

Part III: Bioavailability of metronidazole floating dosage forms.

The aim of the following experimental work is the study of the bioavailability of the chosen prepared formulae of metronidazole as compared to the commercially available metronidazole tablets namely Flagyl, after being orally administered to human volunteers. The pharmacokinetics parameters of different metronidazole treatments administered orally to human volunteers have been calculated. These

16

parameters including C_{max}, t_{max}, k_{ab}, k_{el}, $t_{1/2\,ab}$, $t_{1/2\,el}$, V_d, TCR, AUC $_{0-24}$, $AUC_{24-\infty}$, $AUC_{0-\infty}$, $AUMC_{0-24}$, $AUMC_{\infty-24}$, $AUMC_{0-\infty}$, C_{max}/AUC_{0-24} and MRT. Also, the relative bioavailability of the chosen metronidazole formulae compared to the commercial product was estimated.

The obtained results showed that:

1-Regarding the peak drug plasma concentration, C_{max}, the investigated treatments can be arrangend, in a descending manner, as follows: metronidazole tablet containing Carbopol 934 with ratio 2:1 (formula 3tA), metronidazole tablet containing methyl cellulose with ratio 2:1 (formula 7tA), metronidazole tablet containing CMC with ratio 1:1 (formula 5tB), metronidazole capsule containing pectin with ratio 1:2 (formula 8cD), and metronidazole capsule containing HPMC 15000 with ratio 2:3 (formula 1cC). In other terms, metronidazole tablets containing Carbopol 934 with ratio 2:1 (formula 3tA) has the highest rate and extent of drug absorption concerning the oral treatments estimated.

2-The time necessary to reach a maximum peak concentration, t_{max}, which reflects the rate of drug absorption, was found to be 4 hours for metronidazole tablet containing Carbopol 934 in drug: polymer ratio 2:1, one hour for metronidazole tablet containing CMC in drug: polymer ratio 1:1, 2 hours for metronidazole tablets prepared with methyl cellulose in drug: polymer ratio 2:1, 3 hours for both metronidazole capsule containing HPMC 15000 in drug: polymer ratio 2:3and metronidazole capsule containing pectin in drug: polymer ratio 1:2.

3-The maximum $AUC_{0-\infty}$have been showed with formula 3tA (tablets containing CMC in ratio 1:1) and measured 244.604 µg.hr/ml, while the minimum $AUC_{0-\infty}$ was belonging to formula 1cC (capsules containing HPMC 15000 in ratio 2:3) and was 5.988541 µg.hr/ml.

4-Regarding the area under plasma concentration time curve, $AUC_{0-\infty}$, which reflects the bioavailability, the investigated treatments can be arranged, in descending manner, as follows: metronidazole tablets containing CMC in ratio 1:1, metronidazole tablets containing methyl cellulose in ratio 2:1, metronidazole tablets containing Carbopol 934 with ratio 2:1, metronidazole capsules containing pectin in ratio 1:2, and metronidazole capsules containing HPMC 15000 in ratio 2:3.

5-Regarding the mean residence time of metronidazole formulae, MRT, can be arranged in a descending manner, as follows: metronidazole tablets containing CMC in ratio 1:1, metronidazole tablets containing methyl cellulose in ratio 2:1 , metronidazole capsules containing pectin in ratio 1:2, metronidazole capsules containing HPMC 15000 in ratio 2:3 and metronidazole tablets containing Carbopol 934 with ratio 2:1.

6-According to the absorption rate constant, K_{ab}, the investigated treatments can be arranged, in a descending order, as following: metronidazole tablets containing CMC in ratio 1:1 (formula 5tB), metronidazole capsule containing HPMC 15000 in ratio 2:3 (formula 1cC), metronidazole tablets containing Carbopol 934 in ratio 2:1 (formula 3tA), metronidazole capsules containing pectin in ratio 1:2 (formula 8cD), and metronidazole tablets containing methyl cellulose in ratio 2:1 (formula 7tA).

7-The elimination rate constant, k_{el}, of the investigated treatments can be arranged, in a descending order, as follows: metronidazole tablets containing methyl cellulose with ratio 2:1 (formula 7tA), metronidazole tablets containing Carbopol 934 with ratio 2:1 (formula3tA), metronidazole capsules containing HPMC 15000 with ratio 2:3 (formula1cC), metronidazole capsules containing pectin with ratio 1:2 (formula 8cD), and metronidazole tablets containing CMC with ratio 1:1 (formula5tB).

8-Regarding the percentage relative bioavailability of metronidazole treatments to standard commercial tablets (RB), the investigated treatments can be arranged, in a descending order, as follows: metronidazole tablets containing CMC in ratio 1:1(formula 5tB), metronidazole tablets containing methyl cellulose in ratio 2:1 (formula 7tA), metronidazole tablets containing Carbopol 934 in ratio 2:1 (formula 3tA), metronidazole capsules containing pectin in ratio 1:2 (formula 8cD), and metronidazole capsules containing HPMC 15000 in ratio 2:3 (formula 1cC).

Formula 5tB which is metronidazole tablets containing CMC in drug: polymer ratio 1:1 was found to be the best studied treatment as it showed short t_{max}, medium C_{max}, medium MRT, good K_{ab}, and the best relative bioavailability.

INTRODUCTION

Introduction

The site specific delivery of drugs to target receptor sites has the potential to reduce effects and to increase pharmaceutical response.

The goal of any drug delivery system is to provide a therapeutic amount of drug to the proper site in the body to achieve promptly, and then maintain, the desired drug concentration.

In recent years, there has been increased interest in the development and marketing of prolonged action or controlled release drug delivery systems. Some drugs are inherently long-lasting and require only once-a-day oral dosing to sustain adequate drug blood levels and the desired therapeutic effect. These drugs are formulated in the conventional manner in immediate-release dosage forms. However, many other drugs are not inherently long-lasting and require multiple daily dosing to achieve the desired therapeutic effect.

Multiple daily dosing often is inconvenient for the patient and can result in missed doses, made-up doses and patient noncompliance with the therapeutic regimen. When conventional immediate release dosage forms are taken on schedule and more than once daily, there are sequential therapeutic blood level peaks and valleys (troughs) associated with the taken of each dose Figure (1a).

However, when doses are not administered on schedule, the resulting peaks and valleys reflect less than optimum drug therapy. For Example, if doses are administered too frequently, minimum toxic concentrations (MTC) of drug may be reached with toxic side effects

21

resulting. If doses are missed, periods of sub therapeutic drug blood levels or those below the minimum effective concentration (MEC) may result with no patient benefit.

Extended-release tablets and capsules are commonly taken only once or twice daily compared with counterpart conventional forms that may need to be taken three to four times daily to achieve the same therapeutic effect. Typically, extended-release products provide an immediate release of drug which promptly produces the desired therapeutic effect which when then is followed by the gradual and continual release of additional amounts of drug to maintain this effect over a predetermined period of time Figure (1b). The sustained plasma drug levels provided by extended –release drug products often times eliminates the need for night dosing, which provides benefit not only to the patient but to the caregiver as well (Rogers and Kwan, 1979) (Bogner, 1997) (Madan, 1985a).

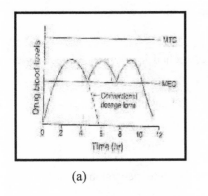   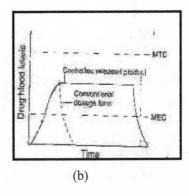

(a)   (b)

Figure (1): Hypothetical drug blood   level-time curves for a conventional solid dosage form: (a) a multiple-action product. (b) a controlled release product.

Some advantages of extended-release systems are given in Table (1). Some disadvantages are the loss of flexibility in adjusting the drug dose and/or dosage regimen, and an increased risk of sudden and total drug release or "dose dumping" due to failure of the technology of the dosage unit.

Drug products that provide "extended" or "sustained" drug release first appeared as a major new class of dosage form in the late 1940s and early 1950s (Madan, 1985b). Over the years, many terms (and abbreviations) as sustained release (SR), sustained action (SA), prolonged action (PA), controlled release (CR), extended release (ER), timed release (TR), and long acting (LA), have been used by manufacturers to describe product types and features . Although these terms often have been used interchangeably, individual products bearing these descriptions may differ in design and performance and must be examined individually to ascertain their respective features. For the most part, these terms are used to describe orally administered dosage forms, whereas the term rate-controlled delivery is applied to certain types or drug delivery systems in which the rate of drug delivery is controlled by features of the device rather than by physiological or environmental conditions as gastrointestinal pH or drug transit time through the gastrointestinal tract.

Modified-release.

In recent years, this term has come into general use to describe dosage forms having drug release features based on time, course, and/or location which are designed to accomplish therapeutic or convenience objectives not offered by conventional or immediate-release forms (Bogner, 1997) (AAPS/FDA, 1995) . The USP differentiates modified-release forms as extended-release and delayed-release (USP, 2000).

23

Extended release

The FDA defines an extended-release dosage form as one that allows a reduction in dosing frequency to that presented by a conventional dosage form, e.g., a solution or an immediate-release dosage form (Bogner, 1997).

Delayed-release

A delayed-release dosage form is designed to release the drug from the dosage form at a time other than promptly after administration. The delay may be time-based or based on the influence of environmental conditions, as gastrointestinal pH (Ansel et al., 1999).

Repeat Action

These forms usually contain two single doses of medication, one for immediate release and the second for delayed release. Bilayered tablets, for example, may be prepared with one layer of drug for immediate release with the second layer designed to release drug later as either a second dose or in an extended-release manner (Ansel et al., 1999).

Targeted Release

Targeted release describes drug release directed toward isolating or concentrating drug in a body region, tissue or site for absorption or for drug action (Ansel et al., 1999).

Table (1): Advantages of Extended-Release Dosage forms over conventional forms.

Advantage	Explanation
Reduction in drug blood level fluctuations	By controlling the rate of drug release, "peaks and valleys" of drug-blood levels are eliminated.
Frequency reduction in dosing	Extended-release products deliver frequently more than a single dose of medication and thus they may be taken less often than conventional forms.
Enhanced patient convenience and compliance	With less frequency of dose administration, a patient is less apt to neglect taking a dose. There is also greater patient and/or caregiver convenience with daytime and nighttime medication administration.
Reduction in adverse side effects	Because there are fewer drug blood level peaks outside of the drug's therapeutic range and into the toxic range adverse side effects occur less frequently.
Reduction in overall health care costs	Although the initial cost of extended release dosage forms may be greater than that for conventional dosage forms the overall cost of treatment may be less due to enhanced therapeutic benefit, fewer side-effects, and reduced time required of health care personnel to dispense and administer drugs and monitor patients.

Extended –Release Oral Dosage Forms

Not all drugs are suited for formulation into extended-release products and not all medical conditions require treatment with such a product. The drug and the therapeutic indication must be considered jointly in determining whether or not to develop an extended-release dosage form (Ansel et al., 1999).

For a successful extended-release product, the drug must be released from the dosage form at a predetermined rate, dissolve in the gastrointestinal fluids, maintain sufficient gastrointestinal residence time, and be absorbed at a rate that will replace the amount, of drug being metaobolized and excreted.

In general, the drugs best suited for incorporation into an extended release product have the following characteristics.

They exhibit neither very slow nor very fast notes of absorption and excretion. Drugs with slow rates of absorption and excretion are usually inherently long acting and their preparation into extended release dosage forms is not necessary. Drugs with very short half lives, i.e., <2 hours, are poor candidates for extended release dosage forms because of the large quantities of drug required for such a formulation. It should also be noted that drugs which act by affecting enzyme systems may be longer acting than indicated by their quantitative half-lives due to residual effects and recovery of the diminished biosystem (Madan, 1990).

They are uniformly absorbed from the gastrointestinal tract. Drugs prepared in extended release forms, must have good aqueous solubility and maintain adequate residence time in the gastrointestinal tract (Ansel et al., 1999).

26

They are administered in relatively small doses. Drugs with large single doses frequently are not suitable for the preparation of an extended release product because the oral dosage unit (tablet or capsule) needed to maintain a sustained therapeutic blood level of the drug would have to be too large for the patient to easily swallow (Ansel et al., 1999).

They possess a good margin of safety. The most widely used measure of the margin of a drug's safety is its therapeutic index. i.e., the median toxic dose divided by the median effective dose.

For very "potent" drugs the therapeutic index may be "narrow" or very small. The larger the therapeutic index, the safer the drug. Drugs which are administered in very small doses or possess very narrow therapeutic indices are poor candidates for formulation into extended release formulation because of technologic limitations of precise control over release rates and the risk of dose "dumping" due to a product defect. Patient misuse (e.g., chewing dosage unit) also could result in toxic drug levels (Ansel et al., 1999).

They are used in the treatment of chronic rather than acute conditions. Drugs for acute conditions require greater physician adjustment of the dosage than that provided by extended-release products (Ansel et al., 1999).

However, the design of an oral controlled drug delivery system is precluded by several physiological difficulties, such as an inability to restrain and localize the drug delivery system within desired regions of the gastrointestinal tract (GIT) and the highly variable nature of gastric emptying process.

Gastric emptying of dosage forms is an extremely variable process, and the ability to prolong and control the emptying time would be a valuable asset in the delivery of certain therapeutic agents. Drugs released from devices that achieve gastric retention would be emptied with the gastric contents over a prolonged period and would thus be present at the main absorption site, the small intestine, for a longer time. This prolonged gastric retention could improve bioavailability and reduce drug wastage.

One group of drugs that would benefit from retentive formulation is those that are absorbed in a relatively narrow region in the proximal part of the GIT (Roug et al., 1996). Once a dosage form passes beyond this region, any further drug release is essentially wasted. Examples of such drugs are furosemide (Chungi et al., 1979), cyclosporine (Drewe et al., 1992), allopurinol (Schuster et al., 1985), and ciprofloxacin (Harder et al., 1990).

Drugs that are less soluble in the higher pH environment of the small intestine than in the stomach may also benefit from gastric retention. This would reduce the possibility of dissolution becoming the rate limiting step in release from dosage form. Examples are weak bases drug such as chlordiazepoxide (Sheth and Tossounian 1984) and Cinnarizine (Machida et al., 1989) .A similar situation would be the formulation of a drug such as captopril (Matharu & Sanghavi 1992) that is degraded by the pH conditions of the small intestine.

28

One reason for wishing to prolong the gastric retention of a dosage form is to achieve a local therapeutic effect. Although there is uncertainty as to whether the antibacterials used to eradicate Helicobacter pylori from the stomach act locally or systemically (Cooreman et a., 1993), there is evidence to show that prolonged local concentration of antibacterials may be of value in achieving eradication of Helicobacter pylori infections (Burton et al., 1995) (Patel and Amiji 1996) (Cremer, 1997). Similarly, Oth et al., 1992 devised a system for the local delivery of misoprostil, a cytoprotectant, to enhance activity for the prevention and treatment of non steroidal anti-inflammatory agent damage.

1-Anatomical and physiological considerations in the design of oral modified-release formulations (floating dosage forms):

1.1-Anatomy of the stomach:

The stomach is anatomically divided into three parts: fundus, body, and antrum (or pylorus). The proximal stomach, made up of the fundus and body regions, serves as a reservoir for ingested materials while the distal region (antrum) is the major site of mixing motions, acting as a pump to accomplish gastric emptying (Desai, 1984) Figure (2).

1.2-Physiology of Gastric Emptying:

The process of gastric emptying occurs both during fasting and fed states; however, the pattern of motility differs markedly in the two states. In the fasted state, it is characterized by an interdigestive series of electrical events which cycle both through the stomach and small intestine every 2-3 hours (Fell, 1996)

29

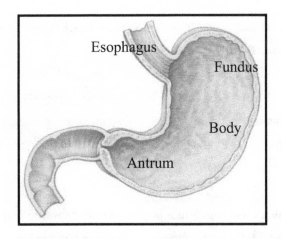

Figure (2): Anatomy of the stomach. Adopted from (Desai, 1984)

This activity is described by Wilson and Washington, 1989, phase I is a quiescent period lasting from 40 to 60 minutes with rare contractions. Phase II is a period of similar duration consisting of intermittent action potentials and contractions that gradually increase in intensity and frequency as the phase progress. Phase III is a short period of intense, large regular contractions lasting from 4 to 6 minutes. This phase, gives the cycle of "housekeeper" wave, where it sweeps the undigested materials out of the stomach and down the small intestine. Phase IV is a brief transitional phase that occurs between phase III and phase I of two consecutive cycles .In the fed state, the gastric emptying rate is slowed since the onset of migrating myoelectric cycle (MMC) is delayed (Desai, and Bolton, 1993).

In the fed state, the stomach handles liquids and solid materials in different ways (Hinder and Kelly 1977) (Siegal et al., 1988) (Horowitz et al., 1989). Liquids are emptied first (usually within 30 minutes) by slow and sustained contractions of the proximal stomach (Gupta and Robinson, 1988) (Mojaverian et al., 1991).

The gastric emptying time of a solid meal depend on the type (weiner et al., 1981) (lin et al., 1990), nutrition density (Hunt and stubbs, 1975), Quantity, and particle size of the meal (Davis et al., 1984).It can be extended to over 14 hour if fed state conditions are maintained (Mojaverian et al., 1985).

Particles less than 5 mm in diameter are known to emptied by the contractions of the distal stomach following the emptying of liquids. Emptying of the solid digestible food particles longer than 5 mm is delayed until they are reduced in size by the grinding action of the stomach (Kelly, 1981). Indigestible solids larger than 5 mm in diameter are retained within the stomach until the digestive process is complete. The gastric emptying time for a regular meal is about 2-6 hours (Chien, 1992).The emptying of large indigestible objects from the stomach is dependent on the contraction activity of the indendigestive migrating motor complex (IMMC)(Kelly 1981) (Minami et al., 1984) (Itoh et al., 1986).

Scintigraphic studies involving measurements of gastric emptying rates in healthy human subjects have revealed that an orally administered controlled release dosage form is mainly subject to two physiological adversities, the short gastric residence time (GRT) and the variable (unpredictable) gastric emptying time (GET). Yet another major adversity encountered through the oral route is the first pass effects, which lead to reduced systemic bioavailability of a large number of drugs. These problems can be exacerbated by alteration in gastric emptying that occur due to factors such as age, race, sex, and disease states, as they may

31

seriously affect the release of a drug from the drug delivery systems. It is therefore, desirable to have a controlled release product that exhibits an extended GI residence and a drug release profile independent of patient related variables (Brahma and Kwon, 2000).

1.3-Factors affecting gastric retention:

Perhaps the greatest challenge in design of oral modified release formulations and the establishment of useful in vitro-in vivo correlations is the changing nature of the gastro intestinal tract from the stomach to the Colon (Lipka, and Amidon, 1999).

There are several factors that can affect gastric emptying (and hence gastric residence time) of an oral dosage form. These factors include density size, and shape of dosage form, concomitant intake of food and drugs such as anticholonergic agents (e.g., atropine), opiates (e.g., Codeine), and biological factors such as gender, posture, age, body mass index, and disease states (e.g., diabetes, Crohn's disease).

Floating drug delivery systems are retained in the stomach for a prolonged period of time by virtue of their floating properties, which can be acquired by several means. Generally speaking, in order for such system to float in the stomach the density of the dosage form should be less than the gastric contents. A density of less than 1.0 g/ml has been reported in the literatures.

While considering the role of specific gravity in gastric residence time, the potential of food in modifying gastric residence should not be overlooked. One of the earlier in vivo evaluations of floating drug delivery systems by Muller – Lissner and Blum, 1981, demonstrated that a gastric residence time of 4-10 hours could be achieved after a fat and protein test meal.

Further-more, food affects the gastric residence time of dosage forms depending on its nature, caloric content and the frequency of intake (Oth et al., 1992) (Moore et al., 1984) (Mojaverian et al 1985). Iannuccelli et al., 1998, reported that in the fed state after a single meal, all the floating units has a floating time (FT) of about 5 hours and a gastric residence time prolonged by about 2 hours over the control. Obviously, when the gastroretentive properties of a floating dosage form are independent of meal size, it can be suggested that the dosage form will be suitable for patients with a wide range of eating habits (Whitehead et al., 1998).

Interestingly, most of the studies related to effects of food on gastric residence time of floating drug delivery system share a common viewpoint that food intake is the main determinant of gastric emptying, while specific gravity has only a minor effect on the emptying process (Davis et al., 1986 (Mazer et al., 1988) (Sangekar et al., 1987) (Muller-lissner, and Blum 1981).

In fact, studies have shown that the gastric emptying times for both floating and non-floating single units are significantly prolonged after a meal (around 4hours) (Davis et al., 1986) (Muller – lissner, and Blum 1981) (Agyilirah et al., 1991). Moreover, in the fasted stomach the amount of liquid is not sufficient for the drug delivery buoyancy and the stomach's entire contents are emptied down the small intestine within 2-3 hours because of the typical phase III activity (Rubinstein and Friend, 1994).

For instance studies have shown that the of gastric residence time of a dosage form in the fed state can be also influenced by its size (Oth et al., 1992).

Timmermans et al., 1989 studied the effect of size on the gastric residence time of floating and non-floating units. They found that floating units with a diameter equal to or less than 7.5 mm had longer gastric residence times compared to non-floating units.

The prolongation of the gastric residence time by food is expected to maximize drug absorption from floating drug delivery system. This may be rationalized in terms of increased dissolution of drug and longer residence at the most favorable site of absorption. The effects of food on various aspects of drug absorption have been extensively discussed by singh, 1999.

A part from food and buoyancy effects, there are other biological factors that can influence the gastric residence time. Mojaverian et al., 1988 investigated the effects of gender, posture, and age on the gastric residence time. As a result of this study, the mean gastric residence time in the males was significantly faster than in their age and race matched female counterparts. In the case of elderly, the gastric residence time was prolonged, especially in subjects >70 years old.

Another confounding factor is the variability of gastric intestinal tract transit within and between individuals. Studies by Coupe et al., 1991 revealed that variability in the gastric emptying of single and multiple unit systems was large compared to that in small intestinal transit times. However the intra-subject variation was less than inter-subject for both gastric and small intestinal transit times.

34

A comparative evaluation of the gastric transit of floating and non-floating matrix dosage forms indicated that buoyancy and non-buoyancy of the forms lead to distinct intragastric behaviors (Timmermans, 1990).It was also concluded that depending on the subject posture, either standing or supine, the gastric residence period of a dosage form is function of either its buoyancy or the diametric size of the matrix (Van Gansbeke et al., 1991).

In upright subjects, all the floating forms stayed continuously above the gastric contents irrespective of their size, whereas the non-floating units sank rapidly after ingestion .Moreover, in supine subjects, a size effect influenced the gastric residence time of both the floating and non-floating forms. Bennett et al., 1984 have demonstrated the rate of posture in gastric emptying. They observed that an alginates raft emptied faster than food in subject lying on their left side or on their backs and slower in subjects lying on their right side with the raft positioned in the greater curvature of the stomach. This is because when the subjects laid on their left side, the raft was presented to the pylorus ahead of meal and so emptied faster (Wilson and Washington, 1989).

2-Previous studies on Gastric Retention Devices: (Approaches to gastric retention):

Several different approaches have been developed to achieve extended gastric residence time of oral drug delivery system. This particular topic was recently reviewed by Hwang et al., 1998.

2.1-Food Excipient Method:

In corporation of passage – delaying food excipients, especially fatty acids, can extend the gastric emptying time (Groning and Heun, 1984) (Palin et al., 1982). More than 2 hours gastric residence time was achieved in the fasted state when triethanolamine myristate was used as excipient (Groning and Heun, 1982).

2.2-Floating Devices:

Floating dosage forms have a bulk density lower than that of gastric fluids and therefore, are expected to remain buoyant on the stomach contents to prolong the gastric retention time (Sheth and Tossoun lan, 1984) (Thanoo et al., 1993) (Bolton and Desai, 1989) (Deshpande et al., 1997) (Timmermans and Moes, 1990) (Deshpande et al., 1996). For the floating dosage forms to be effective, however, large amounts of water have to be present in stomach all time. Since, as mentioned before, the stomach empties liquids very quickly (within 30 minutes), these floating devices will not be effective without continuous drinking of large quantities of water.

Floating single-unite dosage forms, also called hydrodynamically balanced systems, have been extensively studied (Singh and Kim 2000).

These single-unit dosage forms have the disadvantages of a release all-or-nothing emptying process (kaniwa et al., 1988). However, the multiple- unit particulate dosage forms pass through the gastro intestinal tract to avoid the vagaries of gastric emptying and thus release the drugs more uniformly. The uniform distribution of these multiunit dosage forms along the gastro intestinal tract could result in more reproducible drug absorption and reduced risk of local irritation than the use of single-unit

36

dosage forms (Galeone et al., 1981). Surprisingly however, less attention has been focused on the development of floating microspheres, (Kawashima et al., 1991) (Kawashima et al., 1992) (Thanoo et al., 1993) (Jayanthi et al., 1995).

2.3- High-Density dosage forms:

Bechgaard and Ladefoged 1978, attempted to prolong the gastric retention time by the use of high-density pellets. This is accomplished by coating the drug with a heavy inert material such as barium sulfate, zinc oxide, titanium dioxide and iron powder. They reported that for ileostomy subjects the average transit time for light and heavy pellets from mouth to ileostomy bag were 7 and 25 hours respectively. However, more recent studies by the same group showed that such differences did not exist Bechgaard et al., 1985.

2.4- Mucoadhesive dosage forms:

These dosage forms are based on the adhesive capacities of some polymers with mucins covering the surface epithelium of the stomach (Lenaerts and Gurny, 1990). For examples, polycarbophil or crosslinked poly acrylic acid (Park and Robinson, 1984) (Park and Robison 1985) and a hydrophobic protein called zein (Mathiowitz et al., 1994) were used to design formulations that can adhere to the stomach lining for the extended gastric retention. The main weakness of this approach is that the mucoadhesive can be easily contaminated by the soluble mucins and other proteins present in the gastric juice. This leads to loss of their adhesive capacity to the stomach lining.

However, there are some inherent problems associated with such systems since they will deliver a large amount of drug at a particular site

37

of the gastro intestinal tract, thereby leading to local irritation (Chang et al., 1985).

2.5- Dosage forms with special shapes:

Cargill et al., 1988 reported certain shape elastomers or plastics made from polyethylene or nylon could increase the gastric retention time. Tetrahedrons and rings provided gastric retention longer than 24 hour. These dosage forms, however, were neither digestible nor easy to load and release drugs (Caldwell et al., 1988a) (Cald well et al., 1988b) (Fix et al., 1993) (kedzierewicz et al., 1999).

2.6- Magnetic dosage forms:

"Magnetic tablets" were made by mixing ferrite powder with other excipients (Fujimori et al., 1994) (Fujimori et al., 1995).After administration; these tablets were retained in the stomach by an externally applied strong magnetic field. The strong external magnetic field, however, is not readily available in practical use.

2.7- Balloon devices:

Michaels et al., 1975 developed a device that compromised a collapsed envelope containing a liquid, such as, n-pentane, converting to a gas at body temperature. The device can expand to a size larger than the pyloric canal for retention in the stomach. In stead of low boiling point organic solvents, osmotic agents can be used to inflate the envelope (Mamajek and Moyer, 1980) .This approach, while effective, is not easy implement.

2.8- Highly swelling hydrogel dosage forms:

Hydrogels can be retained in the stomach by swelling to a size larger than of the pyloric canal (shalaby et al., 1992a) (Shalaby et al., 1992 b) (Urquhart and Theeuwes, 1984). Although a hydrogel can swell to hundreds of times its dried size, its swelling is very slow. It takes several hours before it reaches a size larger enough to be retained in the stomach. Because the Cyclic IMMC (indigestive migrating motor complex) movement occurs every 2 hours, the hydrogel is most likely to be expelled from the stomach before it swells to a required size. Thus, hydrogels should possess a fast swelling property to be useful as a gastric retention device.

3-synthesis and developments of floating drug delivery system (FDDS)

The concept of floating drug delivery system was described in the literature as early as 1968.When Davis disclosed a method for over coming the difficulty experienced by some persons of gagging or choking while swallowing medicinal pills. He suggested that such difficulty could be overcome by providing pills having a density of less than 1g/ml so that pill will float on water surface. Since then several approaches have been used to develop an ideal floating delivery system.

The various buoyant preparations include hollow microspheres (microballoons), granules, powder, capsules, tablets (pills), and laminated films. A list of drug used in the development of floating drug delivery system (FDDS) thus far is given in Table (2, 3).

Based on the mechanism of buoyancy, two distinctly different systems have been utilized in the development of floating drug delivery

39

system (FDDS). The various approaches used in and their mechanism of buoyancy are discussed in the following subsections.

3.1-Non effervescent floating drug delivery system (FDDS):

One of the approaches to the formulation of such floating dosage forms involves intimate mixing of drug with a gel-forming hydrocolloid, which swells in contact with gastric fluid after oral administration and maintains a relative integrity of shape and bulk density of less than unity within the outer gelatinous barrier (Hilton and Deasy, 1992).

The most commonly used excipients in non effervescent floating drug delivery system (FDDS) are gel- forming or highly swellable cellulose type hydrocolloids, polysaccharides, and matrix forming polymer such as polycarbonate, polyacrylate, polymethacrylat and polystyrene.

The air trapped by the swollen polymer confers buoyancy to these dosage forms. In addition, the gel structure acts as a reservoir for sustained drug release since drug is slowly released by a controlled diffusion through the gelatinous barrier (Sheth and Tossounian, 1984).

The working principle of the hydrodynamically balanced system (HBS) is more clearly illustrated in Figure (3).

Sheath and Tossounian 1978 developed a hydrodynamically balanced system (HBS) capsule containing a mixture of a drug and hydrocolloids. Upon contact with gastric fluid, the capsule shell dissolves; the mixture swells and forms a gelatinous barrier thereby remaining buoyant in the gastric juice for an extended period of time.

40

Desai and Bolton 1993, 1989, developed controlled release floating tablets of theophylline using agar and light mineral oil. Tablets were made by dispersing a drug/mineral oil mixture in a worm agar gel solution and pouring the resultant mixture into tablet molds, which on cooling and air drying formed floatable controlled release tablets.

Gupta 1987 developed floating ampicillin tablets. However, the formula included a buffer system that was expected to improve the stability of ampicillin in acidic medium, especially in the slow release tablets .In this study, sodium citrate was used as a buffering agent, which maintained a pH of about 6.0 in the microenvironment of ampicillin molecules in the tablets.

Dennis et al., 1992, described a buoyant controlled release powder formulation, which may be either filled into capsules or compressed into tablets. The formulation was considered unique in the sense that it released the drug at a controlled rate regardless of the pH of the environment, being free of calcium ion and CO_2 producing material, and had drug release properties similar to a tablet of identical composition. Other authors, have also prepared tablets with alginate and HPMC that were able to float on gastric contents and provided sustained release characteristics (Davis et al., 1986) (Muller-lissner et al., 1981) (Sheth and Tossounian 1984).

Both the desired time period for buoyancy and the rate of drug release can be modulated by the appropriate selection of a polymer matrix .Polymers such as polycarbonate has been used to develop hollow microspheres that were capable of floating on the gastric fluid and released their drug contents for prolonged period of time.

41

Two types of alginate gel beads capable of floating in the gastric cavity were prepared by Murata et al., 2000. The first, alginate gel bead containing vegetable oil (ALGO), is a hydrogel bead and its buoyancy is attributed to vegetable oil held in the alginate gel matrix. The model drug, metronidazole, contained in ALGO was released gradually into artificial gastric juice, the release rate being inversely related to the percentage of oil. The second, alginate gel bead containing chitosan (ALCS), is a dried gel bead with dispersed chitosan in the matrix. When ALCS containing metronidazole was administered orally to guinea pigs, it floated on the gastric juice and released the drug into the stomach. These release properties of alginate gels are applicable not only for sustained release of drugs but also for targeting the gastric mucosa.

The poor bioavailability of orally dosed furosemide is due to the presence of a biological window in the upper gastrointestinal tract. Iannuccelli et al., 2000, developed and optimized in-vitro a multiple-unit floating system with increased gastric residence time for furosemide.. The complete dose release over the actual intragastric residence time of the system (about 8 hours) was achieved by loading both the core and the membrane forming the units with a 1:5 furosemide/polyvinyl pyrrolidone solid dispersion.

Physicochemical analysis suggested the predominant role of the amorphous state of furosemide in producing enhanced drug solubility and dissolution rate, which led to the desired release profile from the floating units.

Table (2): List of drugs explored for various floating dosage forms.

D.f*	DRUG	REFERENCE
Microspheres	Aspirin,griseofulvin, and p-nitroaniline	Thanoo et al., 1993.
	Ibuprofen	Kawashima et al., 1992.
	Terfenadine	Jayanthi et al., 1995.
	Tranilast	Kawashima et al., 1991 and
Granules	Diclofenac sodium	Yuasa et al., 1996.
	Indomethacin	Miyazaki et al., 1988.
	Prednisolone	Inouye et al., 1989.
Films	Cinnarizine	Machida et al., 1989.
Capsules	Chlordiazepeoxide	Sheath and Tossounian 1984.
	Diazepam	Sheath and Tossounian 1984;
	Furosimide	Menon et al., 1994.
	Misoprostol	Franz and Oth, 1993; Oth et al.,
	Propranolol	Khattar et al., 1990.
Tablets pills	Acetaminophen	Phuapradit, 1989; Phuapradit and
	Acetosalicylic acid	Sheth and Tossounian, 1979.
	Amoxycililin	Hilton and Deasy, 1992.
	Ampicillin	Gupta, 1987.
	Atenolol	Rouge et al., 1998 a and b.
	Theophylline	Desai and Bolton, 1993 b;Yange and
	Verapamil HCl	Asrani, 1994.
	Piretanide	Rouge et al., 1998 b.
	Sotalol	Chueh et al., 1995.

*D.f (dosage form).

Table (3): Comparison of GRTs of floating and non- floating solid dosage forms.

| Drugs | Dosage forms | GRT (hour) | | References |
		NFDS	FDDS	
Diazepam	Capsules	1-1.5	4-10	Sheth and Tossounian, 1984.
Ethmozine	Tablets	1-1.5	>6	Regmi et al.,1996.
Gentamycine sulfate	Tablets	1-2	>4	Xu et al., 1991.
Isradipine	Capsules	0.51-2.87	2.4-4.8	Mazer et al., 1988.
Metoprolol tartrate	Tablets	1-1.5	5-6	Li et al., 1989.
Miocamycin	Tablets	3-4	>7	Diao and Tu,1991.
Pepstatin	Minicapsules	NR	3-5	Umezawa, 1978.
Salbutamol sulfate	Capsules	NR	8-9	Babu and aKhar, 1990
Tranilast	Microballoons	NR	>3	Kawashima et al., 1991.

GRT (gastric residence time); NFDS (non-floating delivery system) FDDS (floating drug delivery system); NR (not reported).

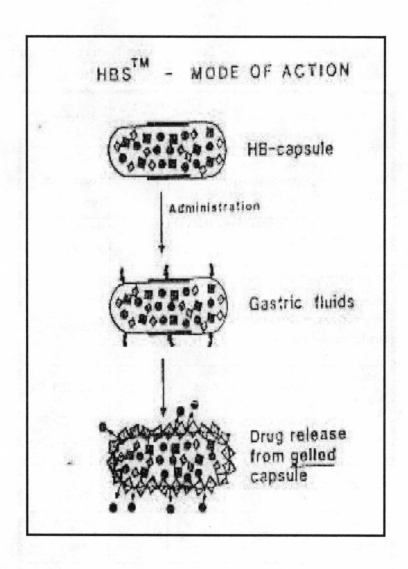

Figure (3): Working principle of the hydrodynamically balanced system (HBS). The hard gelatin capsule contains a special formulation of hydrocolloids, which swell into a gelatinous mass upon contact with gastric fluids. Adopted from Bogentoft (1982).

Bulgarelli et al., 2000, studied the effect of matrix composition and process conditions on casein-gelatin beads floating properties. Casein-gelatin beads have been prepared by emulsification extraction method and cross-linked with D, L-glyceraldhyde in an acetone-water mixture 3:1 (v/v).Casein emulsifying properties cause air bubble incorporation and the formation of large holes in the beads. The high porosity of the matrix influences the bead properties such as drug loading, drug release and floatation. The study shows that cavities act as an air reservoir and enable beads to float. Therefore, casein seems to be a material suitable to the inexpensive formation of an air reservoir for floating systems.

Optimization of floating matrix tablets and evaluation of their gastric residence time have been made by Baumgartner et al., 2000. Tablets containing hydroxypropyl methyl cellulose (HPMC), drug and different additives were compressed. The investigation shows that tablet composition and mechanical strength have the greatest influence on the floating properties and drug release. With the incorporation of a gas-generating agent together with microcrystalline cellulose, besides optimum floating (floating lag time, 30 second; duration of floating, >8 hours), the drug content was also increased.

Xu, and Groves 2001, have studied the effect of FITC-dextran molecular weight on its release from floating cetyl alcohol and HPMC tablets. An anomaly was noted in the release behavior of a series of high molecular weight fluorescein isothiocyanate dextrans (FITC-dextrans) from a tablet formulation designed to float in stomach contents. The tablets contained sodium bicarbonate and hydroxy propyl methylcellulose (HPMC) in a cetyl alcohol matrix. When hydrated in an acid medium, his tablet consisted of a mixed solid with a viscous surface layer containing carbon dioxide bubbles through which the active ingredient (FITC-dextran) was released into the aqueous environment. The key constraint

46

appeared to be the apparent gel pore-size of the hydrated HPMC that was approximately 12 nm in diameter, irrespective of the molecular weight of the HPMC samples evaluated. It was concluded that FITC-dextran release was controlled by both FITC-dextran molecular weight and the HPMC hydrogel structure.

El-Gibaly, 2002 have developed and in-vitro evaluates of novel floating chitosan microcapsules for oral use with comparison with non-floating chitosan microspheres. Floating microcapsules containing melatonin were prepared by the ionic interaction of chitosan and a negatively charged surfactant, sodium dioctyl sulfosuccinate. The characteristics of the floating microcapsules generated compared with the conventional non-floating microspheres manufactured from chitosan and sodium tripolyphosphate were also investigated. The effect of various factors (cross linking time, sodium dioctyl sulfosuccinate and chitosan concentrations, as well as drug/polymer ratio) on microcapsule properties was evaluated. Chitosan concentration and drug/polymer ratio had a remarkable effect on drug entrapment in sodium dioctyl sulfosuccinate/chitosan microcapsules. The release of the drug from these microcapsules was greatly retarded with release lasting for several hours, compared with non-floating microspheres where drug release was almost instant. Most of the hollow microcapsules developed tended to float over simulated biofluids foe more than 12 hours. Therefore, data obtained suggest that the floating hollow microcapsules produced would be an interesting gastro retentive controlled-release delivery system for drugs.

Effect of adding non-volatile oil as a core material for the floating microspheres prepared by emulsion solvent diffusion method have been studied by Lee et al., 2001.Eudragit microspheres, to float in the gastrointestinal tract, were prepared to prolong a gastrointestinal transit

47

time. To enhance their buoyancy, non-volatile oil was added to the dispersed phase. When an oil component was not miscible with water, over 90% was entrapped within the microspheres and prolonged the floating time of the microspheres. Depending on the solvent ratio, the morphologies of the microspheres were different and the best result was obtained when the ratio of dichloromethane: ethanol: isopropanol was 5:6:4. Compared with microspheres prepared without non-volatile oil, the release rate of the drug from microspheres was faster in all cases tested, except the microspheres containing mineral oil. The solubility of the drug in the non-volatile oil affected the release profiles of the drugs. The internal morphology of the microspheres was slightly different depending on the entrapped oil phase used. Tiny spherical objects were present at the inner surface of microspheres and the inside of the shell.

Thanoo et al., 1993 developed drug loaded polycarbonate microspheres using a solvent evaporation method. A high drug loading (>50%) was achieved by this process. Furthermore, increasing the drug to polymer ratio in the microspheres increased their main particle size and the release rate of the drugs.

Kawashima et al., 1991 and 1992, prepared hollow microspheres (microballoons) with drug loaded in their outer shells, by an emulsion – solvent diffusion method. The gas phase generated in the dispersed polymer droplet by the evaporation of dichloromethane formed an internal cavity in the microspheres of the polymer with the drug .During the in-vitro testing, the micro balloons floated continuously over the surface of an aqueous or an acidic dissolution medium for more than 12 hours.

Yuasa et al., 1996 developed intragastric floating and sustained release granules of diclofenac sodium using a polymer solution of HPLC grade, ethyl cellulose and calcium silicate as a floating carrier, which has a characteristically porous structure with numerous pores and a large individual pore volume.

Whitehead et al., 1996 developed a multiple unit floating dosage form from freeze dried calcium alginate. Spherical beads were produced by dropping a sodium alginate solution into aqueous calcium chloride. The results of resultant-weight measurements suggested that these beads maintained a positive floating force for over 12 hours.

Iannuccelli et al., 1998 a and b, described a multiple unit system that contained an air compartment. The units forming the system were composed of a calcium alginate, core separated by an air compartment from a membrane of calcium alginate or calcium alginate/PVA. The in-vitro results suggested that the floating ability increased with an increase in PVA concentration and molecular weight.

Sato et al., 2004 have evaluated the in-vitro and the in-vivo behavior of riboflavin-containing microballoons for floating controlled drug delivery systems in healthy human volunteers. The microballoons possessing a spherical cavity enclosed within a hard polymer shell have been developed as dosage form characterized by excellent buoyancy in the stomach. Microballoons were prepared by the emulsion solvent diffusion method using enteric acrylic polymers dissolved in a mixture of dichloromethane and ethanol. These microballoons were evaluated in vivo by analysis the urinary excretion of riboflavin. The intragastric

49

floating properties of microballoons are potentially beneficial as far as a sustained pharmacological action is concerned.

Sato et al., 2003, developed a hollow microsphere (microballoons) by the emulsion solvent diffusion method utilizing enteric acrylic polymers dissolved in a mixture of dichloromethane and ethanol. Riboflavin powder, riboflavin containing microballoons, and riboflavin containing nonfloating microspheres were administered orally to each of three healthy volunteers. In view of the finding regarding similar riboflavin release profiles of microballoons and nonfloating microspheres in solution of pH 1.2 and solution of pH 6.8, the intragastric floating properties of microballoons appeared be beneficial with respect to sustained pharmacological action.

Streubel et al., 2003a have developed a new preparation method for low density foam-based, floating microparticles and demonstrate the system's performance in-vitro. Major advantages of a novel preparation technique include,(i) short processing times,(ii) no exposure of the ingredients to high temperatures,(iii) the possibility to avoid toxic organic solvents, and (iv) high encapsulation efficiencies close to 100%. Good in -vitro drug release and floating behavior was observed in most cases and a broad variety of drug release patterns could be achieved by varying the drug loading and type of polymer.

Lis et al., 2003, investigate the effect of HPMC and Carbopol on the release and floating properties of gastric floating drug delivery system using factorial design. HPMC of different viscosity grades and Carbopol 934 p were used in formulating the gastric floating drug delivery system employing 2×3 full factorial design. It was found that both HPMC viscosity, the presence of Carbopol and their interaction had significant impact on the release and floating properties of the delivery system. The decrease in the release rate was observed with an increase in the viscosity of the polymeric system.

Streubel et al., 2003b, have developed physicochemically characterize single unit, floating controlled drug delivery systems consisting of polypropylene foam powder, matrix-forming polymers, drug, and filler (optional). The highly porous foam powder provided low-density and, thus excellent in-vitro floating behavior of the tablets. All foam powder-containing tablets remained floating for at least 8 hours in 0.1 N HCl at 37°C. The floating behavior of the low density drug delivery systems could successfully be combined with accurate control of the drug release patterns.

Alginate gel beads containing ethylcellulose were prepared and investigated regard to buoyancy, in-vitro and in-vivo drug release profiles, and drug targeting specificity in the gastric mucosa by Murata et al., 2003. When the ethylcellulose content of alginate gel beads containing metronidazole was higher than 3%, the beads floated in all test solution with a specific gravity of approximately 1.01. Alginate gel beads released metronidazole gradually and floated throughout the experimental period in simulated gastric juice.

Streubel et al., 2002, developed floating microparticles based on low density foam powder. Floating microparticles consisting of propylene foam powder, verapamil hydrochloride as model drug, and Eudragit RS, ethylcellulose or poly methyl methacrylate as polymers were prepared with an o/w solvent evaporation method. Encapsulation efficiencies close to 100% could be achieved by varying either the ratio amount of ingredients. In all cases, good in vitro floating behavior was observed.

51

Joseph et al., 2002 have made in-vitro, in-vivo evaluation of floating-type oral dosage form for piroxicam based on hollow polycarbonate microspheres. A floating type dosage form of piroxicam in hollow polycarbonate microspheres capable of floating on simulated gastric and intestinal fluids was prepared by a solvent evaporation technique. Incorporation efficiencies of over 95% were achieved for the encapsulation. The amount released increased with time for 8 hours after which very little was found to be released up to 24 hours. The data obtained in this study demonstrated that floating dosage form of piroxicam in polycarbonate microspheres was capable of sustained delivery of the drug for longer periods with increased bioavailability.

Soppimath et al., 2001 have developed a hollow microspheres as floating controlled-release systems for cardiovascular drugs. Hollow microspheres of cellulose acetate loaded with four cardiovascular drugs (nifedipine, nicardipine hydrochloride, verapamil hydrochloride, and dipyridamole) were prepared by a novel solvent diffusion-evaporation method. The oil-in-water emulsion prepared in an aqueous solution of 0.05% polyvinyl alcohol medium with ethyl acetate, a water-soluble and less toxic solvent, was used as the dispersion solvent. The yield of the microspheres was up to 80%. The microspheres tended to float over the gastric media for more than 12 hours. The release of the drugs was controlled for more than 8 hours.

El-Kamel et al., 2001 prepared and evaluated ketoprofen floating oral delivery system. A sustained release system for ketoprofen designed to increase its residence time in the stomach without contact with the mucosa was achieved through the preparation of floating microparticles by the emulsion-solvent diffusion technique. For different ratios of

52

Eudragit S 100 with Eudragit RL were used to form the floating microparticles. All floating microparticle formulations showed good flow properties and packability. Release rates were generally low in 0.1 N HCl especially in presence of high content of Eudragit S while in phosphate buffer pH 6.8, high amounts of Eudragit S100 tended to give a higher release rate.

A synergism between a bioadhesive system and a floating system has also been explored. Chitnis et al., 1991 synthesized a series of bioadhesive polymers that were cross- linked polymers of methacyrlic acid and acrylic acid. Floating tablets of isosorbide, mononitrate were prepared and then dipcoated with Carbopol suspensions and finally air dried. The results showed that tablets coated with bioadhesive polymers had better adhesive properties at pH 1.0 as compared to those coated suspensions of Carbopol.

A new strategy based on gastric retention is proposed for the treatment of Helicobacter pylori by Umamaheswari et al., 2002. A synergism between a floating and a bioadhesive system has been explored. Floating microspheres containing the anti-ureas drug acetohydroxamic acid were prepared by anovel quasi-emulsion solvent diffusion method. The microballoons were coated with 2% w/v solution of polycarbophil by the air suspension coating method. The results suggest that acetohydroxamic acid-loaded floating bioadhesive microspheres are superior as potent ureas inhibitors.

Nur,and Zhang 2000 have designed the captopril floating and/ or bioadhesive tablets. Two viscosity grades of hydroxy propyl methyl cellulose (HPMC 4000 and 15, 0000 cps) and Carbopol 934P were used to prepare captopril floating tablets. In vitro dissolution was carried out in simulated gastric fluid at 37°C.Compared to conventional tablets, release of captopril from these floating tablets was apparently prolonged; as a result, a 24-hours controlled release dosage form for captopril was achieved.

3.2- Effervescent floating drug delivery system (FDDS):

These buoyant delivery systems utilize matrices prepared with swellable polymers such as methocel or polysaccharides as chitosan, and effervescent components, e.g., sodium bicarbonate and citric or tartaric acid (Rubinstein and Friend, 1994) or matrices containing chambers of liquid that gasify at body temperature (Ritsch, 1991) (Michaels et al., 1975) (Michaels, 1974) . The matrices are fabricated so that upon arrival in the stomach, carbon dioxide, is liberated by the acidity of gastric contents and is entrapped in the jellified hydrocolloid. A decrease in specific gravity causes the dosage form to float on the chyme (Rubinstein and Friend, 1994).

The carbon dioxide generating components may be intimately mixed within the tablet matrix in which case a single-layered tablet is produced (Hashim and Liwanpo 1987) or a bilayered tablet may be compressed in which contains the gas generating mechanism in one hydrocolloid containing layer and the drug in the other layer formulated for sustained release effect (Ingani et al., 1987).

This concept has also been exploited for floating capsule systems. Stockwell et al., 1986, prepared floating capsules by filling with a mixture of sodium alginate and sodium bicarbonate.

Recently a multiple unit type of floating pill, which generates CO_2 gas, has been developed Ichikawa et al., 1991.The system considered of sustained release pill as seeds surrounded by double layers Figure (4a). The inner layer was an effervescent layer containing both sodium bicarbonate and tartaric acid. The outer layer was a swellable membrane layer containing mainly polyvinyl acetate and purified shellac. When the system was immersed in a buffer solution, it sank at once in the solution and formed swollen pills, like the balloons, with a density much lower than 1g/ml. The reaction was due to co_2 generated by neutralization in the inner effervescent layers with the diffusion of water through the outer swellable membrane layers Figure (4b).

The system was found to float completely in 10 minutes and approximately 80% remained floating over a period of 5 hours irrespective of pH and viscosity of the test medium.

A variant of this approach utilizing citric acid and sodium bicarbonate as effervescing agents and hydroxy propyl cellulose as a release controlling agents has been reported (Watanabe et al., 1993).

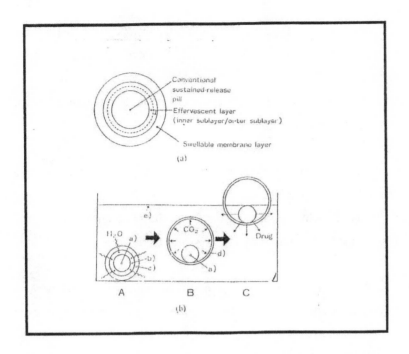

Figure (4): (a) A multiple-unit oral floating dosage system. Reproduced with permission from Ichikawa et al., (1991). (b) Stages of floating mechanism: (A) penetration of water; (B) generation of CO_2 and floating; (C) dissolution of drug. Key(a)conventional SR pills;(b) effervescent layer;(c) swellable layer;(d) expanded swellable membrane layer;(e) surface of water in the beaker.

It is worth mentioning that carbonates in the inner layer of formulation, in addition to imparting buoyancy to this formulation, provide the initial alkaline micro environment for polymers to gel (Deshpande, et al., 1997). Moreover, the release of CO_2 helps to accelerate the hydration of the floating tablets is essential for the formation of a bioadhesive hydrogel (Asrani, 1994).

As a matter of fact, there are several factors that influence the buoyancy of floating tablets. These include nature of excipients, viscosity grades of the polymers, tablets weight, tablet density, tablet diameter and pH of the dissolution medium (Phuapradit, 1989) (Phuapradit and Bolton, 1991) (Gerogiannis et al., 1994).

Similar formulation variables are known to affect the in- vitro performance of floating capsules. These variables include polymer excipients, contents of the polymers, weight of the filled powdered mixture, and the amount of the effervescent added (Chen and Hao, 1998).

Atyabi et al., (1994, 1996 a, b) developed a floating system utilizing ion exchange resins. The system consisted of resin beads, were loaded with bicarbonate and a negatively charged drug that was bound to the resin. The resultant beads were then encapsulated in a semi permeable membrane to overcome rapid loss of CO_2.

Umamaheshwari et al., 2003, have prepared cellulose acetate butyrate-coated cholestyramine microcapsules as an intragastric floating drug delivery system endowed with floating ability due to the carbon dioxide generation when exposed to the gastric fluid. The microcapsules also have a mucoadhesive property. Ion-exchange resin particles can be loaded with bicarbonate followed by acetohydroxamic acid and coated with cellulose acetate butyrate by emulsion solvent evaporation method. The effect of cellulose acetate butyrate: drug-resin ratio on the particle size, floating time, and drug release was determined. The buoyancy time of cellulose acetate butyrate-coated formulations was better than that of uncoated resin particles. These results suggest that cellulose acetate butyrate-coated microcapsules could be a floating as well as

57

mucoadhesive drug delivery system. Thus, it has promise in the treatment of Helicobacter pylori.

Nicardipine hydrochloride, a calcium channel blocker with significant vasodilating and anti hypertensive activities, was formulated as sustained release floating capsules by Moursy et al., 2003. A hydrocolloid of high viscosity grade was used for the floating systems. The inclusion of sodium bicarbonate to allow evolution of carbon dioxide to aid buoyancy was studied. Polymers that retard drug release were included as coprecipitates and granule preparation via wet granulation were used. The hydrocolloid used succeeded in effecting capsule buoyancy. Floating time increased with increasing the proportion of the hydrocolloid. All the seven floating capsule formulae prepared proved efficient in controlling drug release.

Furthermore, the system was capable of slow release of drug, a property which widens the scope of such floating system for sustained release preparation of drugs possessing negative charge since they can be easily bound to the resin in combination with bicarbonate ions. Todd and Fryers 1979, described a similar formulation which contained anhydrous cholestyramine, low viscosity grade alginic acid, sodium alginate, citric acid, and sufficient sodium carbonate or bicarbonate mixtures thereof to neutralize the acid groups of the alginic and citric acid.

Floating dosage forms with an in situ gas generating mechanism are expected to have greater buoyancy and improved drug release characteristics. However, the optimization of the drug release may alter the buoyancy and therefore, it is some times necessary to separate the

58

control of the buoyancy from that of drug release kinetics during formulation optimization (Rouge, 1996).

Choi et al., 2002, prepared alginate beads for floating drug systems and studied the effect of carbon dioxide gas-forming agents. Floating beads were prepared from a sodium alginate solution containing $CaCo_3$ or $NaHCo_3$ as gas-forming agents. The solution was dropped to 1% $CaCl_2$ solution containing 10% acetic acid for carbon dioxide gas and gel formation. As gas-forming agents increased, the size and floating properties increased. The enhanced buoyancy and sustained release properties of $CaCo_3$-containing beads make them an excellent candidate for floating drug dosage systems.

A new kind of two-layer floating tablet for gastric retention with cisapride as a model drug was developed by Wei et al., 2001. Because of the sodium bicarbonate added to the floating layer, when immersed in simulated gastric fluid the tablet expands and rises to the surface, where the drug is gradually released. The in vitro drug release of this kind of two-layer dosage was controlled by the amount of hydroxy propyl methyl cellulose (HPMC) in the drug-loading layer. Generally, the more HPMC, the slower the drug releases.

The development of an optimized gastric floating drug delivery system is described by Li et al., 2001. Statistical experimental design and data analysis using response surface methodology is also illustrated. A central, composite Box-Wilson design for the controlled release of calcium was used with 3 formulation variables: X1 hydroxy propyl methyl cellulose loading, X2 citric acid loading, and X3 magnesium staerate loading. Twenty formulations were prepared, and dissolution

59

studies and floating kinetics were performed on these formulations. Optimization of the formulations was achieved by applying the constrained optimization. The quadratic mathematical model developed could be used to further predict formulation with desirable release and floating properties.

The release kinetics for effervescent floating systems significantly deviates from the classical Higuchi model and approach zero-order kinetics systems (Hashim and Liwanpo, 1987) (Ichikawa et al., 1991) (Chen and Hao, 1998). This deviation in drug release behavior has been attributed to air entrapped in the matrix (Korsmeyer et al., 1983), which is considered a barrier to diffusion, and matrix relaxation (Chen and Hao, 1998). In contrast, non-effervescent floating systems obey the Higuchi model, indicating that drug release occurs via a diffusion mechanism (Desai and Bolton, 1993 b) (Khattar et al., 1990) (Chen and Hao, 1998) (Babu and Khar, 1990).

Li et al., 2002 evaluate the contribution of formulation variables on the floating properties of gastric floating drug delivery system using a continuous floating monitoring system and statistical experimental design. Several formulation variables, such as different types of HPMC, varying HPMC/Carbopol ratio, and addition of magnesium stearte, were evaluated using Taguchi design, and the effects of these variables were subjected to statistical analysis. The statistical analysis indicated that magnesium staerate had a significant effect on the floating property of gastric floating drug delivery system, and addition of magnesium stearate could significantly improve the floating capacity of the gastric floating drug delivery system.

4-Marketed Products of floating drug delivery system (FDDS):

Madopar® HBS is a commercially available product used in Europe and other countries. It contain 100 mg levodopa and 25 mg benserazide, a peripheral dopa decarboxylase inhibitor .This controlled release formulation consists of a gelatin capsule that is designed to float on the surface of the gastric fluids .The drugs diffuse as successively hydrated boundary layers of the matrix dissipate (Erni and Held 1987).

Val-release® is second example of a floating capsule, marketed by Hoffman-La Roche, which contains 15 mg diazepam which is more soluble at low pH. Thus, diazepam absorption is more desirable in the stomach, not in the intestine where it is practically insoluble and is poorly absorbed. The hydrodynamically balanced system (HBS) system maximizes the dissolution of the drug by prolonging the gastric residence time (GRT) (Sheth and Tossounian, 1984).

Floating liquid alginate preparations e.g. liquid Gaviscon, are used to suppress gastroesophageal reflux and alleviate the symptoms of heart burn. The formulation consists of a mixture of alginate, which forms a gel of alginic acid and a carbonate or bicarbonate component which react with gastric acid and evolve Co_2 bubbles. The gel becomes buoyant by entrapping the gas bubbles, and floats on the gastric contents as a viscous layer, which has a higher pH than the gastric contents (Washington et al., 1986).

Topalkan® is a third-generating aluminum magnesium antacid that involves not only its antacid properties but an even greater degree the availability of alginic acid in its formulation (Degtiareva et al., 1994). Almagate Flot-Coat® is another novel antacid formulation that confers a

61

higher antacid potency together with a prolonged gastric residence time and safe as well as extended delivery of antacid drug (Fabregas et al., 1994).

5-Importance of floating drug delivery system (FDDS):
5.1-Sustained drug delivery:

As mentioned earlier, drug absorption from oral controlled release dosage forms is often limited by the short gastric residence time available for absorption. However hydrodynamically balanced system type dosage forms can remain in the stomach for several hours and, therefore, significantly prolong the gastric residence time (GRT) of numerous drugs (Table 3). These special dosage forms are light, relatively large in size and do not easily pass through the pylorus, which has an opening of approximately 0.9-1.9 cm (Deshpande et al., 1997).

It is worth noting here that a prolonged gastric residence time (GRT) is not responsible for the slow absorption of a lipophilic drug such as isradipine that has been achieved with a floating modified release capsule (Mazer et al., 1988). This is because the major portion of drug release from the modified-release capsule took place in the colon rather than in the stomach. However, the assumed prolongation in gastric residence time (GRT) is postulated to cause sustained drug-release behavior (Rubinstein and Friend 1994).

A recent study by a Chinese group indicated that the administration of diltiazem floating tablets twice a day may be more effective compared to normal tablets in controlling the blood pressure of hypertensive patients (Gu et al., 1992). Although there was no significant difference between the two formulations in terms of maximal decrease in systolic

62

and diastolic pressure, the duration of hypotensive effects was longer with floating tablets than that with normal dose. Further, the t $_{1/2}$ and C_{max} were longer and lower for floating tablets than those of normal tablets, respectively; however the two formulations were bioequivalent.

In case of Madopar[®] HBS, the formulation has been shown to release levodopa for up to 8 hours in-vitro, whereas the release from standard Madopar[®] formulation is essentially complete in less than 30 minutes (Erni and Held, 1987). Pharmacokinetic studies in Parkisonian patients and healthy volunteers have also revealed that Madopar[®] HBS behaves as a controlled /slow-release formulation of l-dopa and benserazide (Malcolm et al., 1987) (Crevoisier et al., 1987).

Desai and Bolton 1993 compared the dissolution profiles of floating theophylline controlled release tablet and a commercial sustained release tablet. They found that floating tablets showed a more gradual release of the drug. The initial release rate was found to be comparatively faster with a slower rate after 8 hours. On the other hand, the release rate of Theo-Dur[®] was slower initially but increased later. However, these differences were not statistically significant, and two formulations were regarded as bioequivalent.

5.2-Site specific drug delivery:

A floating dosage form is a feasible approach especially for drugs such as furosemide and riboflavin, which have limited absorption sites in the upper small intestine. In fact, the absorption of furosemide has been found to be site-specific, the stomach being the major site of absorption, followed by the duodenum (Ritschel et al., 1991). This property prompted the development of a monolithic floating dosage form for furosemide

63

which could prolong the gastric residence time (GRT), and thus its bioavailability was increased (Menon et al., 1994).For instance, a significant increase in absolute bioavailability of floating dosage form of furosemide has been obtained, compared to the commercially available tablet (lasix) and enteric product (Lasix long).Furthermore , among these three dosage forms, only the floating dosage form yielded satisfactory in vitro results that were significantly correlated with in-vivo absorption kinetics.The findings of this study were based on a previous postulation that site-specific absorption and longer gastric residence time (GRT) could possibly increase the bioavailability of furosemide (Ritschel et al., 1991).

Similar observation were made by Ichikawa et al., 1991, who found that floating pills containing p-amino benzoic acid, a drug with a limited absorption site in the gasto intestinal tract, had 1.61 times grater AUC than the control pills.

5.3- Local therapeutic effect:

It has become apparent that consumption of non steroidal anti inflammatory drugs (NSAIDs) and stomach colonization by Helicobacter pylori (H. pylori) are the two most common causes of peptic ulcer disease(Graham, 1996) (Rune, 1996) (Blum , 1996) (Logan, 1994) (Inouye et al., 1989). In the United States, peptic ulcer disease affects 10% of population at some point in their lives (NIH Consensus Development panel, 1994).

The prevention and management of non steroidal anti - inflammatory drugs (NSAID) related gastro intestinal complications are well recognized and in many cases successfully treated (Graham,

64

1996).However, the understanding and treatment of H. pylori-induced ulcers are still in progress.

During the early 1980s, Marshall and Warren 1984 for the first time isolated a spiral, ureas-producing, flagellate gram-negative bacterium which was later identified as Helicobacter pylori, accusative factor in the etiology of peptic ulcer disease. H.pylori appears to be responsible for 95% of cases of gastritis and 65% of gastric ulcers (Lee, 1996).

Although most individuals with H. pylori are asymptomatic, there is now convincing evidence that this bacterium is the major etiologic factor in chronic dyspepsia, H. pylori- positive duodenal and gastric ulcers and gastric malignancy (Tytgat, 1996) (Cooreman et al., 1993). Consequently, H. pylori eradication is now recognized to be the correct approach along with conventional therapies in the treatment of the disease. Options that have been considered to treat peptic ulcer disease include taking drug such as antacids, H_2-blockers, antimuscarinics, and proton pump inhibitors and combination therapy for gastritis associated with H. pylori.

The eradication of H. pylori is limited by its unique characteristics. Once acquired, it penetrates the gastric mucus layer and fixes it self to various phospholipids and glycolipids on the epithelial surface, including phosphatidyl ethanolamine (Gold et al., 1993), GM3 ganglioside (Slomiany et al., 1989) and lews antigen (Boren et al., 1993). Therefore, the organism exclusively resides on the luminal surface of the gastric mucosa under the mucus gel layer in the acidic environment of the stomach see Figure (5). The organism is catalase positive, oxidative ureas positive. As a result, urea is broken down into bicarbonate and ammonia, protects the bacterium in the acid medium of stomach (Marshall et al., 1990) and causes gastric epithelial injury (Trie bling et al., 1991).

For effective H.pylori eradication, therapeutic agents have to penetrate the gastric mucus layer to disrupt and inhibit the mechanism of colonization. This required targeted drug delivery within the stomach environment. Although most antibiotics have very low in-vitro minimum inhibitory concentrations against H.pylori (MIC 90 $\leq$ 1 mg/L) (Tytgat, 1994), no single antibiotics has been able to eradicate this organism effectively. In addition, its eradication from patients requires high concentrations of drug be maintained within the gastric mucosa for a long duration (Blaser, 1992).

Currently, a drug, combination namely 'triple therapy' with bismuth salt, metronidazole, and either tetracycline or amoxicillin with healing rates of up to 94% has been success fully used (Blum, 1996) (Heatley, 1992) (Axon, 1991).

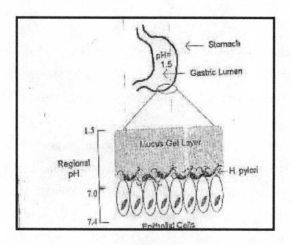

Figure (5): Schematic of H.pylori location within the stomach. The bacteria is S-shaped, gram-negative, having flagella (for more detail, refer to reference Balaban and Peura, 1997).

The principle of triple therapy is to attack H. pylori luminally as well as systemically. The current treatment is based on frequent administration (4 times daily) of individual dosage forms of bismuth, tetracycline, and metronidazole. The associated limitations are the complex dosing regimen, frequency, large amount of dosage forms and reduced patient compliance. Therefore, a successful therapy not only includes the selection of right drugs but also the timing and frequency as well as the formulation of the delivery system.

Libo et al., 1999, proposed a new strategy for the triple drug treatment (tetracycline, metronidazole, bismuth salt) of H.pylori associated peptic ulcers. The bismuth salt will rapidly dissolve while sustained delivery of both tetracycline and metronidazole will follows. The floating feature is incorporated for prolongation of gastric retention time of the delivery system (Ingani et al., 1987) (Timmermans and Moes, 1994) (Erni and Held, 1987) (Moes, 1993), thus increasing localized concentration and effects of the antibiotics.

Recently, katayama et al., 1999 developed SR liquid preparation of ampicillin using sodium alginate that spreads out and adheres to the gastric mucosal surface whereby the drug is continuously released. Thus, it can be expected that topically delivery of a narrow spectrum antibiotic through a floating drug delivery system (FDDS) may result in complete removal of the organisms in the fundal aria of the gastric mucosa due to bactericidal drug levels being reached in this area, and might lead to better treatment of peptic ulcer disease.

Whitehead et al., 2000, described the incorporation of an agent known to be effective against H.pylori, amoxicillin into calcium alginate beads. Drug release studies showed that beads prepared with the amoxicillin solution provided some sustained release characteristics and that there could be improved by the addition of amylose while preparation of the beads from alginate solutions containing the drug in suspension allowed higher drug loadings, at the expense of faster release and lower buoyancy.

An investigation of ongoing effort to develop effective drug delivery systems for the treatment of Helicobacter pylori infection using polycarbonate floating microspheres as drug carrier have been made by Umamaheshwari et al., 2003. In an effort to augment the anti Helicobacter pylori effect of acetohydroxamic acid, floating polycarbonate microspheres which have the ability to reside in the gastrointestinal tract for an extended period, were prepared by emulsion (o/w) solvent evaporation technique. In-vitro studies confirmed the excellent floating properties of polycarbonate microspheres. The drug acetohydroxamic acid and polycarbonate microspheres both showed anti Helicobacter pylori activity in vivo, but the required dose of acetohydroxamic acid was effectively reduced by a factor 10 in the case of polycarbonate microspheres. In conclusion, the floating microspheres more effectively cleared Helicobacter pylori from the gastrointestinal tract than the drug because of the prolonged gastric residence time resulting from the excellent buoyancy of the polycarbonate.

In subsequent section, a complete review on metronidazole is reported as it is a central drug in most regimens of Helicobacter pylori eradication. In order to investigate the previous methods of targeting drug to the stomach as floating drug delivery system.

6-Limitations of floating drug delivery system (FDDS):

One of the disadvantages of floating systems is that they require a sufficiently high level of fluids in the stomach for the drug delivery buoy to float therein and to work sufficiently. However, this limitation can be over come by coating the dosage form with bioadhesive polymers, thereby enabling them to adhere to the mucus lining of the stomach wall (Chitnis et al., 1991). Alternatively, the dosage form may be administered with a glass full of water (200-250 ml). Floating systems are not feasible for those drugs that have solubility or stability problems in gastric fluids. Drugs such as neifedipine, which is well absorbed along the entire gastric intestinal tract and which undergoes significant first-pass metabolism, may not be desirable candidates for floating drug delivery system since the slow gastric emptying may lead to reduced systemic bioavailability (Rouge et al., 1996).Also there are limitations to the applicability of floating drug delivery system for drugs that are irritant to gastric mucosa.

SCOPE OF WORK

In recent years scientific and technological advancements have been made in the research and development of rate-controlled oral drug delivery system by overcoming physiological advertise such as short gastric residence times (GRT), and unpredictable gastric emptying times (GET).

The de novo design of an oral controlled drug delivery system (DDS) should be primarily aimed at achieving more predictable and increased bioavailability of drugs. However, the development process is precluded by several difficulties. It can be anticipated that, depending on the physiological state of the subject and the design of pharmaceutical formulation, the emptying process can last from a few minutes to 12 hours. This variability, in turn, may lead to unpredictable bioavailability and times to achieve peak plasma levels, since the majority of drugs are preferentially absorbed in the upper part of the small intestine (Rouge et al., 1996).

Furthermore, the relatively brief gastric residence time (GRT) in humans, which normally averages 2-3 hours through the major absorption zone (stomach or upper part of the intestine), can result in incomplete drug release from the drug delivery system (DDS) leading to diminished efficacy of the administered dose. Thus, control of placement of a drug delivery system (DDS) in a specific region of the gastrointestinal tract offers numerous advantages especially for drugs exhibiting local action in the proximal gastrointestinal tract or for drugs that degraded in the intestinal fluids. Overall, the contact of the drug delivery system with the absorbing membrane has the potential to maximize drug absorption and may also influence the rate of drug absorption (Longer et al., 1985) (Alvisi et al.,

1996). These considerations have led to the development of oral controlled release (CR) dosage forms possessing gastric retention capabilities.

Several approaches are currently utilized in the prolongation of the gastric residence time, including floating drug delivery systems (FDDS), also known as hydrodynamically balanced systems (HBS).

Since then several approaches have been used to develop an ideal floating delivery system. The various buoyancy preparations include hollow microspheres, granules, powders, and tablets. Based on the mechanism of buoyancy, two distinctly different technologies non-effervescent and effervescent systems have been utilized in the development of floating drug delivery system (FDDS).

Therefore, the aim of this work was the formulation of metronidazole as it has an important role in the treatment of Helicobacter pylori infection of the stomach in different controlled release forms to prolong its duration of action using the floating technique to target the drug into its site of action. In addition, to maintain effective localized concentration of metronidazole and improve patient compliance.

Thus, the experimental work in the present thesis consisted of the following parts:

Part I: **Formulation and In-vitro performance of metronidazole floating dosage forms.**

The experimental work in this part discussed the various approaches of floating and their mechanisms of buoyancy, also study the effect of different polymers with different ratios on the in-vitro release of metronidazole from different preparations (tablets, capsules, and hollow microspheres).Physical tests have been made for the preparation of dosage forms individually.

The kinetic parameters for the in-vitro release of metronidazole were determined in order to explain the mechanism of drug release. Specific program was used for this purpose zero-, first- and second-order kinetics, as well as, controlled diffusion model, Hixson-Crowell cube root law, and Baker and Lonsdale equation were tried.

Accordingly, this part comprises of two chapters as follow:
Chapter I: Effervescent metronidazole floating tablets.
Chapter II: Non-Effervescent metronidazole floating preparations.

Part II: **Accelerated stability of metronidazole floating dosage forms.**

This part, investigates the stability of various metronidazole floating dosage forms which previously gave the best floating time and in-vitro release results in chapter I at two elevated temperatures 35°C and 45°C for 6 months. By applying some form of Arrhenius equation and substituting the experimentally established specific rate constants at the used two elevated temperatures, the energy of activation (Ea) and the decomposition reaction rate constant at room temperature (k_{20}) can be determined. Also, t ½ and t $_{90}$ for each formula can be estimated.

A special computer program was used to determine the kinetic treatment and kinetic parameters of the stability of the investigated metronidazole dosage forms. Zero-, first- and second-order kinetic were tried to choose the most suitable order for stability study.

Part III: **Bioavailability of metronidazole floating dosage forms.**

In this part, the bioavailability of metronidazole of the selected floating dosage forms as compared to commercially available non-floating tablets namely Flagyl after being orally administered to six human volunteers has been discussed. The pharmacokinetics parameters of different metronidazole treatments administered orally to human volunteers include C_{max}, t_{max}, k_{ab}, k_{el}, t $_{1/2ab}$, t $_{1/2\ el}$, V_d, TCR, AUC $_{0-24}$, AUMC $_{0-24}$, AUMC$_{0-\infty}$ and MRT were determined. Also, the relative bioavailability of the selected metronidazole dosage forms compared to the commercial product was estimated.

Part I

FORMULATION AND IN-VITRO PERFORMANCE OF METRONIDAZOLE FLOATING DOSAGE FORMS

Introduction

The term, controlled release and sustained release are not new to those who are working in various disciplines of pharmaceutical research and development (Chien, 1983).

Controlled release drug administration means not only prolonged duration of drug delivery, as in sustained release and prolonged release, but also, implies predictability and reproducibility of drug release kinetics (Chien, 1983).

All of the controlled release drug delivery system will have only limited utilization in the oral controlled administration of drugs as the systems can not remain in the vicinity of the absorption site for the life-time of the drug delivery (Chien, 1983). Therefore, sustained release formulation systems are only suitable for drugs that show no difference in the absorption characters along the whole alimentary canal.

It has become apparent that consumption of nonsteroidal anti-inflammatory drugs (NSAIDs) and stomach colonization by Helicobacter pylori (H.pylori) are the two most common cause of peptic ulcer disease (Graham et al., 1996; Rune, 1996; Blum, 1996; Logan, 1994; and Inouye et al., 1989). The prevention and management of NSAIDs related gastrointestinal complications are well recognized and in many cases successfully treated (Graham et al., 1996).

On the other hand, H.pylori appears to be responsible for about 95% of the cases of gastritis and about 65% of gastric ulcers (Lee, 1996).So,

76

prolonging the gastric residence of a dosage form may be of therapy value. One reason for wishing to prolong the gastric retention of a dosage is to achieve a local therapeutic effect. Although there is uncertainty as to whether the antibacterial used to eradicate H.pylori from the stomach act locally or systemically (Coorenman et al., 1993), there is evidence to show that prolonged local concentration of antibacterial agent as metronidazole, tetracycline and amoxicillin may be of value in achieving eradication. Therefore, a successful therapy not only includes the selection of the right drugs but also the timing and frequency as well as the formulation of the delivery system.

For the following instance, it has been suggested that an active material should be formulated in the form of an hydrodynamically balanced system to enhance its bioavailability: (a) being effective locally in the stomach, (b) having dissolution and or stability problems in the fluids of the small intestine, and (c) being absorbed only in the stomach and or upper part of the small intestine (Sheth and Tossounian 1984).

It has been reported that metronidazole, the active material used in the present study, has a local effect in the therapy of Helicobacter pylori associated gastric ulcers (Blum 1996, Heatley 1992, Axon 1991). So a complete review of metronidazole will be shown in subsequent section.

Metronidazole

Metronidazole is a nitroimidazole antibiotic with limited spectrum of activity. It is active against various protozoa and most gram-negative and gram-positive anaerobic bacteria. It appears to be selective through producing cytotoxic effects in anaerobes by a reduction reaction. The complete mode of action of metronidazole has not been fully elucidated (Freeman et al., 1997; AMA, 1983).

a. Therapeutic uses

Metronidazole is effective for the prevention and treatment of antibiotic-associated pseudomembranous colitis, with 99% of strains inhibited by 4ug/ml or less (Dzink and Bartlett, 1980). It has shown promise in the treatment of Crohn's disease, particularly in patients with colonic and perineal disease (Prantera et al., 1998; Hanauer, 1996).

It is consider the drug of choice for treating entamoebapolecki infections and guinea worm infections (Anon, 1995).

Metronidazole is approved as curative agent in many diseases: in abscess of lung and brain, which caused by bacteroide species (Giron and Ozoktay, 1984). It is also effective in treating amebic enterocolitis (Chowcat and Wyllie, 1976), skin and skin structure infections (Pierleoni, 1984), intra-abdominal infections (Tyburski et al., 1998), and lower respiratory tract infections including pneumonia due to bacteroides species (Tally et al., 1975; Zimmerman et al., 1980).

Metronidazole is effectively used in the treatment of gingival hyperplasia (Wong et al., 1994) and in combination with amoxicilin in duodenal ulcers associated with helicobacter pylori infections (Hoffman et al., 1999; lee et al., 1998).

Topical metronidazole is effective alone (Lowe et al., 1989) or with other antibiotics (Dahi et al., 1998) in the treatment of acne rosacea.

b. Physico-chemical properties of metronidazole.

Metronidazole

Figure (6): Chemical structure of metronidazole.

Metronidazole is a synthetic 1-(2-hydroxyethyl)-2-methyl-5-nitroimidazole. Its empirical formula is $C_6H_9N_3O_3$ and its molecular weight is 171.16 (Martindale, 1993). It is described according to USP (2000) and B.P (1993) as white to pale yellow, odorless crystals or crystalline powder. It darkens on exposure to light. Metronidazole is sparingly soluble in water and in alcohol; slightly soluble in chloroform and in ether and should be protected from light (USP, 2000).

 c. Pharmacokinetics:

Metronidazole is readily absorbed following oral administration. Bioavilability approaches 100% (Ralph, 1983) for orally administered

79

forms, while from the rectal route it is in the range of 59% to 94 %(Kortelainen et al 1982; Tanner et al 1980; Ford et al 1980). Absorption from vaginal route has been reported to be poor (2%) (Cumingham et al., 1994). Absorption and hence metronidazole bioavailability may be delayed, but are not reduced by administration with food (Prod.Info.Flagyl, 1999).

Metronidazole is widely distributed in most body tissues and fluids. It appears in cerebrospinal fluid (Bennett et al., 1994), bronchial secretions (Braga, 1991), bile (Sattar et al., 1982; Nagar et al, 1989), pancreatic tissue (Freeman et al., 1997), and saliva (Amon et al., 1983), and achieves concentrations similar to those in plasma. It also crosses the placenta and rapidly enters the fetal circulation (Freeman et al., 1997). No more than 20% is bound to plasma proteins and volume of distribution is about 0.25 to 0.85 liters/kg (Bennett et al., 1994).

Peak serum levels of 6, 12, 21.4, and 40 ug/ml were achieved in average of 1 to 2 hour after single oral doses of 250, 500, 750, and 2000 mg metronidazole, respectively (Fredericsson et al., 1987; Ralph et al., 1974; Wood&Monro, 1975). While in case of rectal route, it takes 3 hours to be established (Ioannides et al., 1981) and 8 to 12 hours for topical preparations (Prod.Info.Noritate R, 1999).

Metronidazole is metabolized in the liver by side-chain oxidation and glucuronide formation. The principal oxidative metabolites are the hydroxy metabolite (Gjerloff and Arndd, 1982; Wheeler et al., 1978; Stambaugh et al., 1968) which possesses some biological activity (30% to 65%) of the activity of metronidazole (Freeman et al., 1997; Gjerloff and Arnold, 1982) and acetic acid metabolite that has virtually no antibacterial activity (Gjerloff and Arnold, 1982; Wheeler et al, 1978).

Approximately 6% to 18%of metronidazole is excreted in the urine as unchanged drug. The hydroxy metabolite is entirely excreted in the urine (Freeman et al., 1997), with renal clearence about 10 to 11 ml/min (Ralph et al., 1974). Metronidazole is also excreted in breast milk in concentration approaching those in serum following therapeutic doses. Although no toxic effects on the infant have been observed during breast-feeding, the drug should be avoided if possible (Passmore, 1988; Heisterberg and Branebjerg, 1983).

The elimination half-life of parent compound is 6 to 14 hours (Bennett et al., 1994; Jensen and Gugler, 1983), while its hydroxy metabolite is approximately 9.7 hours (Houghton et al, 1979). Half-life may reach up to 34 hours in patients with total renal failure (Houghton et al., 1985).

d. Contraindications

Metronidazole is contraindicated in the first trimester of pregnancy and in patients with hypersensitivity to any nitroimidazole derivatives including metronidazole itself (Martindale, 1993).

e. Adverse Reactions

The adverse effects of metronidazole are generally dose related. The most common are gastro-intestinal disturbances, especially nausea and unpleasant metallic taste (Katz, 1976; Anon, 1976). There have been rare reports of pseudomembranous colitis associated with metronidazole (Bingley and Harding, 1987).

Peripheral neuropathy and epileptiform seizures are serious adverse effects on the nervous system that have been associated especially with high doses of metronidazole or prolonged treatment (Dreger et al., 1998; Boyce et al., 1990).

Temporary moderate leucopenia may occur in some patients receiving metronidazole (Smith, 1980; Walton, 1974).

Other side effects include urethral discomfort (AMA, 1983), darkening of the urine (Bruce, 1971), raised liver enzymes values (Hestin et al., 1994). Acute visual loss has occasionally been reported (Allroggen et al., 2000).

Various attempts have been made to develop floating systems to control drug release; among them is the so-called hydrodynamically balanced system (HBS) (Sheth and Tossounian, 1979; Chien, 1983). Such system is useful for drugs acting locally in the proximal part of gastrointestinal tract or for drugs that degrade in the intestinal fluid; metronidazole is one drug from the former category.

The objective of this part is to develop a new floatable drug delivery system for controlled delivery of metronidazole which is a drug commonly used in eradication of Helicobacter pylori infection. The floating features are incorporated for possible prolongation of the gastric retention time of the delivery system (Ingani et al., 1987; Timmermans and Moes 1994; Erni and Held 1987; Moes 1993), thus increasing localized concentration and effects of the antibiotic.

The principal of buoyant preparation offers a simple and practical approach to not only achieve increased gastric residence time for the dosage form but also modify the drug-release profile (Sheth and Tossounian 1984). The present part outlines systemic approaches for the in vitro preparations development and optimization for enhancing the local effect of metronidazole in stomach.

Several approaches of floating have been studied to develop an ideal floating delivery system in order to prolong the gastric retention of the deliver system. Based on the mechanism of buoyancy, two distinctly different technologies have been utilized in the development of floating drug delivery system, first effervescent system showed in tablet dosage form and second non-effervescent system with capsules dosage form as well as microspheres (microballoons).

The in vitro release of metronidazole from the different dosage forms prepared with different ratios of various polymers as well as the approaches used in their mechanism of buoyancy are discussed in the following part. The kinetic parameters for the in-vitro release of metronidazole were determined and analyzed in order to explain the mechanism of drug release. Specific computer program was used for this purpose.

CHAPTER I

EFFERVESCENT
METRONIDAZOLE FLOATING
TABLETS

Introduction

In recent years scientific and technological developments have been made in the research and development of rate-controlled oral drug delivery systems by overcoming physiological advertise, such as short gastric residence times (GRT). Several approaches are currently utilized in the prolongation of the gastric residence time, including floating drug delivery system (FDDS), also known as hydrodynamically balanced systems (HBS).

Based on the mechanism of buoyancy of floating system, two distinctly different technologies, effervescent and non effervescent systems, have been utilized in the development of floating drug delivery systems (FDDS).

In this chapter, the current technological developments of floating drug delivery system including effervescent floating system were discussed. These buoyant delivery systems include a gas-generating component in the formulation. The gas is then trapped in gellified hydrocolloid to achieve the desired low density. Carbonate or bicarbonate usually include in the formulation, which reacts either with the stomach acid or acid present in the formulation to produce carbon dioxide. The gas-generating system may be part of the complete formulation or may consist of a separate layer.

The present chapter includes formulation, dissolutions, and buoyancy of sustained release tablet of metronidazole then preparation of floating bilayer compressed tablets which is applied for formulae that gave best result of sustained action of metronidazole (be able to deliver the drug at constant rates up to 90% of the total loading dose).

85

For comparison, immediate release reference tablets containing the same dose of metronidazole (plain tablet) but without any polymer were also formulated.

The prepared conventional slow-release tablets of metronidazole were evaluated for their uniformity of weight, thickness, hardness, friability, drug content and disintegration time. The kinetic parameters for the in-vitro release of metronidazole were determined and analyzed in order to explain the mechanism of drug release. Specific computer program was used for this purpose.

Experimental

Material:

- Metronidazole powder, kindly supplied by Egyptian International Pharmaceutical Industries Company (E.I.P.I.Co), Egypt.

- Microcrystalline cellulose (Avicel pH 101), Pectin (USP), Aerosil 200, starch 1500, kindly supplied by El-Nile Pharmaceutical-Chemical Company, Cairo, Egypt.

- Methyl cellulose, Hydroxypropyl methylcellulose (HPMC 4000 and 15000 cps) grades, Na alginate, Carbopol 934, and carboxymethylcellulose (CMC), kindly supplied by El-Kahira Pharmaceutical-Chemical Company, Cairo, Egypt.

- Hydrochloric acid, specific gravity 1.16 GPR, El-Nasr chemicals company, Cairo, Egypt.

- Ethyl cellulose, Fluka (Switzerland).

- Na bicarbonate and calcium carbonate, El-Nasr Chemicals Company, Cairo, Egypt.

Equipment:

- Electric balance: Mettler, J100, (Switzerland).

- Tablet compression machine: Type EV:o. Erweka Apparatus, Frankfurt, (Germany).

- Tablet Thickness Apparatus, Planimeter, (India).

• Digital Tablet Friability Apparatus, (model; FT-2D) VEEGO, Progressive instruments, Bombay, (India).

• Tablet Hardness Tester: Model: TH-16, (China).

• Spectrophotometer, Jenway LTD: Model: 610 suvlvis, (England).

• Modified USP dissolution tester (Scientific). DA.6D, Bombay-400-069, (India).

Methodology:

1-Construction of the standard calibration curve of metronidazole:

The following steps were followed:

1-A stock solution of 0.5 mg/ml was prepared by dissolving 50 mg of metronidazole in 100 ml of 0.1 N HCl pH 1.2.

2- Serial concentrations of 20, 10, 9, 8, 7, 6 and 5ug/ml of metronidazole in 0.1 N HCl pH 1.2 were prepared by diluting the appropriate volumes of the stock solution in 25 ml volumetric flask.

3- The prepared samples were measured spectrophotometrically at 278 nm against 0.1 N HCl pH 1.2 as a blank.

4- According to the data shown in Table (4), the standard calibrating curve Figure (7) was obtained by plotting the absorbance against the concentrations of the prepared metronidazole solutions. The resulting relation was found to obey Beer Lambert's law.

2-Preparation of Metronidazole Tablet

a- Preparation of Conventional Sustained-release metronidazole tablets:

Tables (5 a and b) represent the proposed sustained formulae of metronidazole tablets. The calculated amount of metronidazole, polymers, and additives for each formula were weighed and blended for 10 minutes using drum mixer. Erweka Tablet compression machine with concave faced single punches was used for the manufacture of tablets each of 12 mm in diameter and 500 mg in weight.

Metronidazole: polymer (HPMC 15000, HPMC 4000, Na alginate, Carbopol 934, Pectin, Ethyl cellulose, Methyl cellulose and CMC) in ratios of 2:1, 1:1, 2:3 and 1:2, metronidazole: polymer (HPMC 15000 and Carbopol 934) ratios of 3:1 and 4:1 and metronidazole: polymer (Pectin) ratio 1:3 were used primarily to formulate the sustained release of metronidazole. Aerosil was used in concentration of 1% w/w as a lubricant. Avicel was used as diluent in sufficient quantities to give tablet of 500 mg in weight.

Minimum of 200 tablets were prepared from each formula and the tablets were evaluated. Plain tablets devoid from any polymers were also prepared using the same previous method. The produced formulae that gave best in-vitro result of sustained action of metronidazole (be able to deliver the drug at constant rates up to 90% of the total loading dose) will subjected to the following section.

b- Preparation of bilayer floating metronidazole tablets:

The preparation of the two-layer floating tablet of metronidazole had two steps. First for the conventional slow-release layer, in which the calculated amount of metronidazole, polymer, and additives for the formulae that gave best in-vitro slow release results were weighed and blended for 10 minutes using drum mixer. Second for the gas generating layer, which consisted of 140 mg of Hydroxypropyl methyl cellulose (HPMC 4000) and mixture of sodium bicarbonate: calcium carbonate (1:2 ratio) were weighed and blended. The bilayer tablets were produced using Erweka Tablet compression machine with 12 mm diameter concave faced single punch. The powder mix of each layer was transferred into the die manually, the first and second layer were compressed.

To determine and optimize the floating lag time and buoyancy duration of the delivery system, 7.5, 15, 22.5, 30, 37.5, 45, 52.5 and 60 mg gas generating salt mixtures were incorporated into the gas generating layer while the weight of other formulation components were kept constant.

The relationships between the amount of gas generating salt blends and the buoyancy lag time as well as the duration of system buoyancy are shown in Tables (74 and 75) and illustrated in Figures (25 and 26) respectively.

3-In-vitro release of metronidazole tablets

The release of metronidazole from the prepared conventional slow-release metronidazole tablets was determined by the USP rotating paddle method (type II). The dissolution media consisted of 900 ml simulated gastric fluid (pH 1.2) maintained at 37±0.5°C and the rotation in each vessel was adjusted to be 50 rotation per minute.

One tablet of each formulated metronidazole sustained release system (each contains 125 mg metronidazole) was placed in each of the three dissolution vessels. In addition, the dissolution profile of the plain metronidazole tablets (metronidazole 125mg without addition of polymers) was determined.

Sample of 5ml at specified time intervals was withdrawn from each of the six dissolution media and filtered off. Clear sample was withdrawn from each filtrate and measured spectrophotometrically at 278 nm against the corresponding blank. The dissolution volume was kept constant all over the dissolution time, by compensation of the withdrawn volume.

The percentage metronidazole release was calculated and the mean of three experiments was determined. Mean results were tabulated and graphically illustrated in Tables (54, 56, 58, 60, 62, 64, 66, 68, 70, 71, 72, and 73) and Figures (13-24). The dissolution data were also subjected to a computerized kinetic calculations program. Results are shown in Tables (55, 57, 59, 61, 63, 65, 67, and 69).

4- Floating time and properties of metronidazole bilayer tablets.

USP dissolution apparatus was used in this test (type I). Each of the six glass vessels of the apparatus was filled with 900 ml of simulated gastric fluid of pH 1.2 and all maintained at 37±0.5°C. Each formula of metronidazole tablets that gave best sustained release results was tested separately. The time between the introduction of the dosage form into the dissolution medium and its buoyancy to the top of dissolution medium was taken as buoyancy lag time, and the duration of floating was observed visually and tabulated in Tables (74 and 75) , and illustrated in Figures (25 and 26).

5-Charactarizations of the conventional sustained-release metronidazole tablets

The produced conventional slow-release tablets of metronidazole tablets were evaluated for uniformity of weight, uniformity of thickness, drug content uniformity, hardness, friability and disintegration time.

5.1-Uniformity of weight:

The uniformity of weight was carried out for the prepared tablets according to USP 2000. Twenty tablets from each formula were weighed individually to the nearest 0.1 mg, and the average weight, standard deviation and coefficient of variation percent were calculated. Results are shown in Tables (6, 12, 18, 24, 30, 36, 42, and 48).

5.2-Uniformity of thickness:

The thickness of prepared tablets was measured using Tablet thickness Apparatus (planimeter). The mean thickness, standard deviation and coefficient of variation percent for each formula were calculated. Results are shown in Tables (7, 13, 19, 25, 31, 37, 43, and 49).

5.3-Uniformity of drug content:

According to USP 2000, ten tablets from each formula were assayed individually. The mean drug content percent, standard deviation and coefficient of variation percent were calculated. Results are shown in Tables (8, 14, 20, 26, 32, 38, 44, and 50).

Assay method:

Each tablet was weighed, powdered and levigated with 100 ml diluted hydrochloric acid (1 ml in 100 ml H_2O) in 250 ml volumetric flask. Shake the content for 30 minutes, then complete with diluted hydrochloric acid and filtered. The filtrate was diluted quantitively with diluted hydrochloric acid, to obtain a solution having a concentration of about 0.2 mg of metronidazole/ ml. Ten ml of this solution was transferred into a 100 ml volumetric flask, diluted with dilute hydrochloric acid to volume, and mixed. Concomitantly the absorbance of this test solution was measured spectrophotometrically and that of similarly prepared standard solution, at the maximum absorbance of 278 nm using dilute hydrochloric acid as blank. Percentage drug content, standard deviation and coefficient of variation were calculated. Results are shown in Tables (8, 14, 20, 26, 32, 38, 44, and 50).

5.4-Hardness:

Pharma Test Hardness tester was used. Twenty tablets from each formula were randomly sampled and tested for hardness. The mean hardness, standard deviation and coefficient of variation percent were calculated. Results are shown in Tables (9, 15, 21, 27, 33, 39, 45, and 51).

93

5.5-Friability:

Digital tablet friability tester was used. Ten tablets from each formula randomly sampled were brushed to free from adhering dust using a soft Camel's hairbrush. They were accurately weighed and placed in the drum. The front plate was applied to the drum, and was rotated for a time period of five minutes (100 rotations). At the end of rotation period, the tablets were removed from the drum, carefully brushed to free from adhering dust and weighed. The percent loss of weight was taken as the measure of friability. The test was repeated five times and the mean friability, standard deviation and coefficient of variation percent were calculated. Results are shown in Tables (10, 16, 22, 28, 34, 40, 46, and 52).

5.6-Disintegration test:

Disintegration studies were carried out according to the procedure in the USP 2000. One tablet from each formula was placed in each of the six tubes of the basket and the apparatus was operated, using water maintained at $37\pm0.5°C$ as the immersion fluid. Results are shown in Tables (11, 17, 23, 29, 35, 41, 47, and 53).

Table (4): Relation between metronidazole concentrations and absorbance at 278 nm in 0.1 N HCl pH 1.2.

Concentration ug/ml	Absorbance
5	0.188
6	0.223
7	0.257
8	0.293
9	0.330
10	0.382
20	0.732

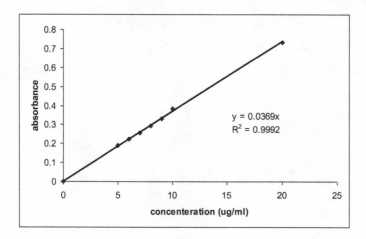

Figure (7): The Beer-Lambert plot for metronidazole in 0.1 N HCl at 278 nm.

Table (5a): Formulation of metronidazole tablets using different polymers with different ratios.

Formula	Formula by weight in mg						
	metronida zole	Avicel pH 101	Aerosil 200	HPMC 15000	HPMC 4000	Carbopol 934	Na alginate
Plain tablet	125	375	5	---	---	---	---
1tA	125	307.5	5	62.5	---	---	---
1tB	125	245	5	125	---	---	---
1tC	125	182.5	5	187.5	---	---	---
1tD	125	120	5	250	---	---	---
1tE	125	328.3	5	41.7	---	---	---
1tF	125	338.75	5	31.25	---	---	---
2tA	125	307.5	5	---	62.5	---	---
2tB	125	245	5	---	125	---	---
2tC	125	182.5	5	---	187.5	---	---
2tD	125	120	5	---	250	---	---
3tA	125	307.5	5	---	---	62.5	---
3tB	125	245	5	---	---	125	---
3tC	125	182.5	5	---	---	187.5	---
3tD	125	120	5	---	---	250	---
3tE	125	328.3	5	---	---	41.7	---
3tF	125	338.75	5	---	---	31.25	---
4tA	125	307.5	5	---	---	---	62.5
4tB	125	245	5	---	---	---	125
4tC	125	182.5	5	---	---	---	187.5
4tD	125	120	5	---	---	---	250

t; tablet dosage form
A; drug: polymer ratio 2:1
B; drug: polymer ratio 1:1
C; drug: polymer ratio 2:3
D; drug: polymer ratio 1:2
E; drug: polymer ratio 3:1
F; drug: polymer ratio 4:1

1; HPMC 15000 (hydroxypropyl methyl cellulose)
2; HPMC 4000 (hydroxypropyl methyl cellulose)
3; Carbopol 934
4; Na alginate
plain tablet; the same ingredients without polymer

Table (5b): Formulation of metronidazole tablets using different polymers with different ratios

Formula	Formula by weight in mg						
	metronidazole	Avicel pH 101	Aerosil 200	CMC	Ethyl cellulose	Methyl cellulose	Pectin
5tA	125	307.5	5	62.5	---	---	---
5tB	125	245	5	125	---	---	---
5tC	125	182.5	5	187.5	---	---	---
5tD	125	120	5	250	---	---	---
6tA	125	307.5	5	---	62.5	---	---
6tB	125	245	5	---	125	---	---
6tC	125	182.5	5	---	187.5	---	---
6tD	125	120	5	---	250	---	---
7tA	125	307.5	5	---	---	62.5	---
7tB	125	245	5	---	---	125	---
7tC	125	182.5	5	---	---	187.5	---
7tD	125	120	5	---	---	250	---
8tA	125	307.5	5	---	---	---	62.5
8tB	125	245	5	---	---	---	125
8tC	125	182.5	5	---	---	---	187.5
8tD	125	120	5	---	---	---	250
8tG	125	---	5	---	---	---	375

t; tablet dosage form
A; drug: polymer ratio 2:1
B; drug: polymer ratio 1:1
C; drug: polymer ratio 2:3
D; drug: polymer ratio 1:2
G; drug: polymer ratio 1:3

5; CMC (carboxy methyl cellulose)
6; Ethyl cellulose
7; Methyl cellulose
8; Pectin

Table (6): Uniformity of weight of metronidazole tablets prepared with different ratios of HPMC 15000.

Formula	Weight (mg)		Standard deviation	Coefficient of variation %
	mean	range		
1tA	504	494-510	7.2	1.40
1tB	501	495-510	5.5	1.10
1tC	502	494-511	4.7	0.93
1tD	504	500-510	3.4	0.67
1tE	501	496-509	3.6	0.72
1tF	503	496-511	4.5	0.89

Table (7): Uniformity of thickness of metronidazole tablets prepared wit different ratios of HPMC 15000.

Formula	Thickness (mm)		Standard deviation	Coefficient of variation %
	mean	range		
1tA	3.86	3.7-4.0	0.11	2.90
1tB	3.96	3.7-4.3	0.17	4.30
1tC	4.05	3.7-4.5	0.40	5.20
1tD	3.90	3.8-4.9	0.29	7.40
1tE	4.00	3.9-4.1	0.07	1.75
1tF	3.90	3.8-4.0	0.06	1.50

1; Polymer HPMC 15000   t; tablet dosage form.
A; drug: polymer ratio 2:1   B; drug: polymer ratio 1:1
C; drug: polymer ratio 2:3   D; drug: polymer ratio 1:2
E; drug: polymer ratio 3:1   F; drug: polymer ratio 4:1

Table (8): Uniformity of content of metronidazole tablets prepared with different ratios of HPMC 15000.

Formula	Drug content (%)		Standard deviation	Coefficient of variation %
	mean	range		
1tA	101.4	100-103	1.50	1.50
1tB	102.6	100-104	1.67	1.60
1tC	97.10	95-98	1.20	1.20
1tD	92.90	92.5-93.5	0.36	0.38
1tE	100.0	99-102	1.10	8.90
1tF	91.90	91.4-92	0.30	0.30

Table (9): Hardness values of metronidazole tablets prepared with different ratios of HPMC 15000.

Formula	Hardness (Kg)		Standard deviation	Coefficient of variation %
	mean	range		
1tA	9.96	9.8-10.1	0.11	1.1
1tB	10.14	9.9-10.7	0.30	2.9
1tC	11.10	10-11.6	0.65	5.8
1tD	10.50	10-11.0	0.36	3.4
1tE	6.70	6.1-7.0	0.30	4.5
1tF	9.95	9.8-10.1	0.10	1.0

1; Polymer HPMC 15000   t; tablet dosage form.
A; drug: polymer ratio 2:1   B; drug: polymer ratio 1:1
C; drug: polymer ratio 2:3   D; drug: polymer ratio 1:2
E; drug: polymer ratio 3:1   F; drug: polymer ratio 4:1

Table (10): Friability values of metronidazole tablets prepared with different ratios of HPMC 15000.

| Formula | Friability (%w/w) | | Standard deviation | Coefficient of variation % |
	mean	range		
1tA	0.198	0.19-0.21	0.008	4.0
1tB	0.98	0.95-1.0	0.020	2.0
1tC	0.62	0.55-0.7	0.068	10.9
1tD	0.43	0.4-0.5	0.045	10.5
1tE	0.58	0.55-0.6	0.020	3.4
1tF	0.22	0.2-0.26	0.030	13.6

Table (11): Disintegration times of metronidazole tablets prepared with different ratios of HPMC 15000.

| Formula | Disintegration time (min) | | Standard deviation | Coefficient of variation % |
	mean	range		
1tA	Tablet swell only			
1tB	Tablet swell only			
1tC	Tablet swell only			
1tD	Tablet swell only			
1tE	21.2	20-25	1.9	8.9
1tF	27.5	25-30	2.8	10.2

1; Polymer HPMC 15000   t; tablet dosage form.
A; drug: polymer ratio 2:1   B; drug: polymer ratio 1:1
C; drug: polymer ratio 2:3   D; drug: polymer ratio 1:2
E; drug: polymer ratio 3:1   F; drug: polymer ratio 4:1

Table (12): Uniformity of weight of metronidazole tablets prepared with different ratios of HPMC 4000.

Formula	Weight (mg)		Standard deviation	Coefficient of variation %
	mean	range		
2tA	501	500-505	2.2	0.44
2tB	506	504-511	1.2	0.23
2tC	505	500-509	3.4	0.70
2tD	505.8	500-512	4.4	0.86

Table (13): Uniformity of thickness of metronidazole tablets prepared with different ratios of HPMC 4000.

Formula	Thickness (mm)		Standard deviation	Coefficient of variation %
	mean	range		
2tA	3.96	3.90-4.10	0.08	2.0
2tB	4.20	3.95-4.40	0.17	4.0
2tC	4.20	4.40-4.70	0.10	2.2
2tD	4.30	4.10-4.50	o.11	2.6

2; Polymer HPMC 4000   t; tablet dosage form.

A; drug: polymer ratio 2:1   B; drug: polymer ratio 1:1

C; drug: polymer ratio 2:3   D; drug: polymer ratio 1:2

Table (14): Uniformity of drug content of metronidazole tablets prepared with different ratios of HPMC 4000.

Formula	Drug content (%)		Standard deviation	Coefficient of variation %
	mean	range		
2tA	95.9	95-96.1	0.12	0.12
2tB	101.0	100-103	1.3	1.3
2tC	100.8	100-102	0.80	0.80
2tD	96.0	95-97	0.89	0.90

Table (15): Hardness values of metronidazole tablets prepared with different ratios of HPMC 4000.

Formula	Hardness (Kg)		Standard deviation	Coefficient of variation %
	mean	range		
2tA	5.40	5.0-6.0	0.30	5.5
2tB	6.98	6.9-7.1	0.08	1.1
2tC	9.30	9.0-10	0.35	3.8
2tD	6.50	6.0-7.0	0.38	5.8

2; Polymer HPMC 4000   t; tablet dosage form.

A; drug: polymer ratio 2:1   B; drug: polymer ratio 1:1

C; drug: polymer ratio 2:3   D; drug: polymer ratio 1:2

Table (16): Friability values of metronidazole tablets prepared with different ratios of HPMC 4000.

Formula	Friability (%w/w)		Standard deviation	Coefficient of variation %
	mean	range		
2tA	0.94	0.9-0.96	0.02	2.1
2tB	0.97	0.9-1.1	0.06	6.2
2tC	0.88	0.86-0.9	0.01	1.1
2tD	0.65	0.6-0.68	0.03	4.6

Table (17): disintegration times of metronidazole tablets prepared with different ratios of HPMC 4000.

Formula	Disintegration time (min)		Standard deviation	Coefficient of variation %
	mean	range		
2tA	Tablet swell only			
2tB	Tablet swell only			
2tC	Tablet swell only			
2tD	Tablet swell only			

2; Polymer HPMC 4000   t; tablet dosage form.

A; drug: polymer ratio 2:1   B; drug: polymer ratio 1:1

C; drug: polymer ratio 2:3   D; drug: polymer ratio 1:2

Table (18): Uniformity of weight of metronidazole tablets prepared with different ratios of Carbopol 934.

Formula	Weight (mg)		Standard deviation	Coefficient of variation %
	mean	range		
3tA	505.0	503-508	2.6	0.5.0
3tB	503.0	500-506	2.0	0.4.0
3tC	503.0	502-508	2.0	0.4.0
3tD	507.0	504-509	1.7	0.33
3tE	511.8	510-517	2.5	0.48
3tF	505.4	503-508	2.5	0.49

Table (19): Uniformity of thickness of metronidazole tablets prepared with different ratios of Carbopol 934.

Formula	thickness (mm)		Standard deviation	Coefficient of variation %
	mean	range		
3tA	4.10	4.0-4.2	0.08	1.9
3tB	4.25	4.10-4.4	0.11	2.5
3tC	4.30	4.00-4.6	0.26	6.0
3tD	4.70	4.60-4.9	0.09	1.9
3tE	3.85	3.80-4.0	0.07	1.8
3tF	4.10	4.00-4.2	0.08	1.9

3; Polymer Carbopol 934   t; tablet dosage form.

A; drug: polymer ratio 2:1   B; drug: polymer ratio 1:1

C; drug: polymer ratio 2:3   D; drug: polymer ratio 1:2

E; drug: polymer ratio 3:1   F; drug: polymer ratio 4:1

Table (20): Uniformity of drug content of metronidazole tablets prepared with different ratios of Carbopol 934.

Formula	Drug content (%)		Standard deviation	Coefficient of variation %
	mean	range		
3tA	99.50	98-101	1.30	1.36
3tB	100.4	100-101	0.54	0.50
3tC	100.8	100-102	0.70	0.69
3tD	97.70	97-100	1.10	1.12
3tE	97.80	97-100	1.10	1.12
3tF	100.40	99-102	0.97	0.966

Table (21): Hardness values of metronidazole tablets prepared with different ratios of Carbopol 934.

Formula	Hardness (Kg)		Standard deviation	Coefficient of variation %
	mean	range		
3tA	15.8	15-17.4	0.90	5.7
3tB	13.6	12-15	1.20	8.8
3tC	16.0	15-18	1.15	7.2
3tD	18.6	18-19.5	0.60	3.2
3tE	16.8	15-19	1.30	7.7
3tF	15.3	14-16.5	0.80	5.2

3; Polymer Carbopol 934   t; tablet dosage form.

A; drug: polymer ratio 2:1   B; drug: polymer ratio 1:1

C; drug: polymer ratio 2:3   D; drug: polymer ratio 1:2

E; drug: polymer ratio 3:1   F; drug: polymer ratio 4:1

Table (22): Friability values of metronidazole tablets prepared with different ratios of Carbopol 934.

Formula	Friability (%w/w)		Standard deviation	Coefficient of variation %
	mean	range		
3tA	0.19	0.195-0.2	0.002	1.1
3tB	0.56	0.54-0.58	0.018	3.2
3tC	0.53	0.5-0.56	0.03	5.7
3tD	0.11	0.1-0.12	0.008	7.3
3tE	0.196	0.19-0.2	0.004	2.0
3tF	0.23	0.2-0.25	0.022	9.6

Table (23): Disintegration times of metronidazole tablets prepared with different ratios of Carbopol 934.

Formula	Disintegration time (min)		Standard deviation	Coefficient of variation %
	mean	range		
3tA	Tablet swell only			
3tB	Tablet swell only			
3tC	Tablet swell only			
3tD	Tablet swell only			
3tE	34.3	30-37	2.9	8.50
3tF	26.0	20-30	4.1	15.7

3; Polymer Carbopol 934   t; tablet dosage form.

A; drug: polymer ratio 2:1   B; drug: polymer ratio 1:1

C; drug: polymer ratio 2:3   D; drug: polymer ratio 1:2

E; drug: polymer ratio 3:1   F; drug: polymer ratio 4:1

Table (24): Uniformity of weight of metronidazole tablets prepared with different ratios of Na alginate.

Formula	Weight (mg)		Standard deviation	Coefficient of variation %
	mean	range		
4tA	499.5	495-505	3.6	0.7
4tB	505	500-510	4.2	0.8
4tC	502.8	494-508	4.7	0.9
4tD	505.6	500-510	3.6	0.7

Table (25): Uniformity of thickness of metronidazole tablets prepared with different ratios of Na alginate.

Formula	Thickness (mm)		Standard deviation	Coefficient of variation %
	mean	range		
4tA	3.80	3.7-3.90	0.07	1.84
4tB	3.90	3.85-4.1	0.07	1.79
4tC	4.08	4.0-4.20	0.07	1.70
4tD	3.68	3.6-3.75	0.04	1.10

4; Polymer Na alginate   t; tablet dosage form.

A; drug: polymer ratio 2:1   B; drug: polymer ratio 1:1

C; drug: polymer ratio 2:3   D; drug: polymer ratio 1:2

Table (26): Uniformity of drug content of metronidazole tablets prepared with different ratios of Na alginate.

Formula	Drug content (%)		Standard deviation	Coefficient of variation %
	mean	range		
4tA	99.7	99-100	3.8	3.8
4tB	100.8	99-102	1.3	1.3
4tC	102.2	100-104	1.3	1.3
4tD	99.8	98-101	1.1	1.1

Table (27): Hardness values of metronidazole tablets prepared with different ratios of Na alginate.

Formula	Hardness (Kg)		Standard deviation	Coefficient of variation %
	mean	range		
4tA	6.2	5.9-7	0.38	6.10
4tB	5.5	4.8-6.5	0.70	12.7
4tC	5.8	5.0-7.0	0.77	13.3
4tD	7.7	6.0-9.0	1.20	15.6

4; Polymer Na alginate   t; tablet dosage form.

A; drug: polymer ratio 2:1   B; drug: polymer ratio 1:1

C; drug: polymer ratio 2:3   D; drug: polymer ratio 1:2

Table (28): Friability values of metronidazole tablets prepared with different ratios of Na alginate.

Formula	Friability (%w/w)		Standard deviation	Coefficient of variation %
	mean	range		
4tA	0.960	0.89-1	0.05	5.2
4tB	0.950	0.9-1.1	0.07	7.4
4tC	1.007	0.98-1.1	0.04	3.97
4tD	0.970	0.9-1	0.04	4.0

Table (29): Disintegration times of metronidazole tablets prepared with different ratios of Na alginate.

Formula	Disintegration time (min)		Standard deviation	Coefficient of variation %
	mean	range		
4tA	6.8	5-9	1.6	23.5
4tB	Tablets swell only			
4tC	5.4	4-7	1.0	18.5
4tD	4.3	3-6	1.1	25.6

4; Polymer Na alginate   t; tablet dosage form.

A; drug: polymer ratio 2:1   B; drug: polymer ratio 1:1

C; drug: polymer ratio 2:3   D; drug: polymer ratio 1:2

Table (30): Uniformity of weight of metronidazole tablets prepared with different ratios of CMC.

Formula	Weight (mg)		Standard deviation	Coefficient of variation %
	mean	range		
5tA	508.0	505-511	1.9	0.4
5tB	503.0	500-506	2.3	0.5
5tC	502.0	500-505	1.9	0.4
5tD	504.5	500-508	3.2	0.6

Table (31): Uniformity of thickness of metronidazole tablets prepared with different ratios of CMC.

Formula	Thickness (mm)		Standard deviation	Coefficient of variation %
	mean	range		
5tA	4.17	4.0-4.3	0.12	2.9
5tB	4.04	4.0-4.2	0.07	1.7
5tC	4.10	4.0-4.2	0.09	2.2
5tD	3.90	3.85-4.1	0.07	1.8

5; Polymer CMC   t; tablet dosage form.

A; drug: polymer ratio 2:1   B; drug: polymer ratio 1:1

C; drug: polymer ratio 2:3   D; drug: polymer ratio 1:2

Table (32): Uniformity of drug content of metronidazole tablets prepared with different ratios of CMC.

Formula	Drug content (%)		Standard deviation	Coefficient of variation %
	mean	range		
5tA	97.5	95-100	1.6	1.6
5tB	98.5	98-100	0.8	0.8
5tC	95.8	95-98	1.2	1.3
5tD	95.8	95-99	1.6	1.7

Table (33): Hardness values of metronidazole tablets prepared with different ratios of CMC.

Formula	Hardness (Kg)		Standard deviation	Coefficient of variation %
	mean	range		
5tA	5.5	5-6	0.50	9.1
5tB	9.4	9-10	0.48	5.1
5tC	4.5	4-5	0.38	8.4
5tD	4.9	4-6	0.60	12.2

5; Polymer CMC   t; tablet dosage form.

A; drug: polymer ratio 2:1   B; drug: polymer ratio 1:1

C; drug: polymer ratio 2:3   D; drug: polymer ratio 1:2

Table (34): Friability values of metronidazole tablets prepared with different ratios of CMC.

| Formula | Friability (%w/w) | | Standard deviation | Coefficient of variation % |
	mean	range		
5tA	0.95	0.90-1.0	0.040	4.2
5tB	0.19	0.18-0.2	0.008	4.2
5tC	0.84	0.8-0.9	0.050	5.9
5tD	0.75	0.7-0.8	0.040	5.3

Table (35): Disintegration times of metronidazole tablets prepared with different ratios of CMC.

| Formula | Disintegration time (min) | | Standard deviation | Coefficient of variation % |
	mean	range		
5tA	Tablets swell only			
5tB	Tablets swell only			
5tC	Tablets swell only			
5tD	Tablets swell only			

5; Polymer CMC   t; tablet dosage form.

A; drug: polymer ratio 2:1   B; drug: polymer ratio 1:1

C; drug: polymer ratio 2:3   D; drug: polymer ratio 1:2

Table (36): Uniformity of weight of metronidazole tablets prepared with different ratios of Ethyl cellulose.

Formula	Weight (mg)		Standard deviation	Coefficient of variation %
	mean	range		
6tA	501.4	500-505	1.90	0.40
6tB	505.3	503-509	1.80	0.40
6tC	505.0	500-508	2.70	0.50
6tD	510.8	510-512	0.89	0.17

Table (37): Uniformity of thickness of metronidazole tablets prepared with different ratios of Ethyl cellulose.

Formula	Thickness (mm)		Standard deviation	Coefficient of variation %
	mean	range		
6tA	3.90	3.8-4.1	0.08	2.1
6tB	4.50	4.2-4.7	0.16	3.5
6tC	4.11	4-4.3	0.11	2.7
6tD	4.32	4.3-4.4	0,04	0.9

6; Polymer Ethyl cellulose   t; tablet dosage form.

A; drug: polymer ratio 2:1   B; drug: polymer ratio 1:1

C; drug: polymer ratio 2:3   D; drug: polymer ratio 1:2

Table (38): Uniformity of drug content of metronidazole tablets prepared with different ratios of Ethyl cellulose.

Formula	Drug content (%)		Standard deviation	Coefficient of variation %
	mean	range		
6tA	99.4	98-101	1.1	1.1
6tB	92.8	91-95	1.5	1.6
6tC	94.5	91-96	1.0	1.1
6tD	98.8	97-100	1.3	1.3

Table (39): Hardness values of metronidazole tablets prepared with different ratios of Ethyl cellulose.

Formula	Hardness (Kg)		Standard deviation	Coefficient of variation %
	mean	range		
6tA	6.1	5-7	0.8	13.0
6tB	5.4	4-7	0.97	17.9
6tC	9.3	9-10	0.40	4.30
6tD	5.7	4-8	1.10	19.3

6; Polymer Ethyl cellulose   t; tablet dosage form.

A; drug: polymer ratio 2:1   B; drug: polymer ratio 1:1

C; drug: polymer ratio 2:3   D; drug: polymer ratio 1:2

Table (40): Friability values of metronidazole tablets prepared with different ratios of Ethyl cellulose.

Formula	Friability (%w/w)		Standard deviation	Coefficient of variation %
	mean	range		
6tA	0.70	0.6-0.8	0.07	10
6tB	0.75	0.6-0.85	0.09	12
6tC	0.65	0.5-0.77	0.10	15
6tD	0.90	0.8-0.99	0.07	7.8

Table (41): Disintegration times of metronidazole tablets prepared with different ratios of Ethyl cellulose.

Formula	Disintegration times (min)		Standard deviation	Coefficient of variation %
	mean	range		
6tA	2.75	1-5	1.2	43.6
6tB	4.40	3-5.5	0.8	18.2
6tC	14.0	13-15	1.0	7.0
6tD	4.0	2-6.5	1.4	29.2

6; Polymer Ethyl cellulose   t; tablet dosage form.

A; drug: polymer ratio 2:1   B; drug: polymer ratio 1:1

C; drug: polymer ratio 2:3   D; drug: polymer ratio 1:2

Table (42): Uniformity of weight of metronidazole tablets prepared with different ratios of Methyl cellulose.

Formula	Weight(mg)		Standard deviation	Coefficient of variation %
	mean	range		
7tA	507	503-512	3.1	0.60
7tB	505.5	500-512	4.1	0.80
7tC	505.3	500-509	3.0	0.06
7tD	509	505-511	2.3	0.45

Table (43): Uniformity of thickness of metronidazole tablets prepared with different ratios of Methyl cellulose.

Formula	Thickness (mm)		Standard deviation	Coefficient of variation %
	mean	range		
7tA	3.90	3.80-4.0	0.08	2.1
7tB	3.90	3.85-4.1	0.08	2.1
7tC	4.30	4.0-4.6	0.27	6.3
7tD	3.95	3.80-4.0	0.07	1.8

7; Polymer Methyl cellulose   t; tablet dosage form.

A; drug: polymer ratio 2:1   B; drug: polymer ratio 1:1

C; drug: polymer ratio 2:3   D; drug: polymer ratio 1:2

Table (44): Uniformity of drug content of metronidazole tablets prepared with different ratios of Methyl cellulose.

Formula	Drug content (%)		Standard deviation	Coefficient of variation %
	mean	range		
7tA	100	98-102	1.60	13.1
7tB	94	92-96	1.50	1.60
7tC	99.5	98-101	1.04	1.05
7tD	97.8	95-99	1.40	1.40

Table (45): Hardness values of metronidazole tablets prepared with different ratios of Methyl cellulose.

Formula	Hardness (Kg)		Standard deviation	Coefficient of variation %
	mean	range		
7tA	9.75	9-11	0.8	8.2
7tB	11.5	10.8-12.8	0.8	6.9
7tC	4.5	3-6.6	1.1	24.4
7tD	10	9-11	0.8	8.0

7; Polymer Methyl cellulose   t; tablet dosage form.

A; drug: polymer ratio 2:1   B; drug: polymer ratio 1:1

C; drug: polymer ratio 2:3   D; drug: polymer ratio 1:2

Table (46): Friability values of metronidazole tablets prepared with different ratios of Methyl cellulose.

Formula	Friability (%w/w)		Standard deviation	Coefficient of variation %
	mean	range		
7tA	0.17	0.10-0.2	0.04	23.5
7tB	0.60	0.50-0.7	0.08	13.5
7tC	0.89	0.85-0.95	0.03	3.40
7tD	0.37	0.30-0.4	0.04	10.8

Table (47): Disintegration times of metronidazole tablets prepared with different ratios of Methyl cellulose.

Formula	Disintegration times(min)		Standard deviation	Coefficient of variation %
	mean	range		
7tA	12.2	10-14	1.6	13.1
7tB	17.6	15-20	2.3	13.1
7tC	Tablets swell only			
7tD	Tablets swell only			

7; Polymer Methyl cellulose   t; tablet dosage form.

A; drug: polymer ratio 2:1   B; drug: polymer ratio 1:1

C; drug: polymer ratio 2:3   D; drug: polymer ratio 1:2

Table (48): Uniformity of weight of metronidazole tablets prepared with different ratios of Pectin.

Formula	Weight(mg)		Standard deviation	Coefficient of variation %
	mean	range		
8tA	506	503-511	3.3	0.65
8tB	503.8	500-508	3.0	0.60
8tC	504	501-507	2.3	4.60
8tD	511	505-515	3.4	0.66
8tG	504	500-510	4.4	0.87

Table (49): Uniformity of thickness of metronidazole tablets prepared with different ratios of Pectin.

Formula	Thickness (mm)		Standard deviation	Coefficient of variation %
	mean	range		
8tA	3.90	3.8-4	0.08	2.1
8tB	3.96	3.7-4.2	0.17	4.3
8tC	3.60	3-4.1	0.30	8.3
8tD	4.10	4-4.2	0.09	2.2
8tG	3.60	3.5-3.7	0.06	1.7

8; Polymer Pectin   t; tablet dosage form.

A; drug: polymer ratio 2:1   B; drug: polymer ratio 1:1

C; drug: polymer ratio 2:3   D; drug: polymer ratio 1:2

G; drug: polymer ratio 1:3

Table (50): Uniformity of drug content of metronidazole tablets prepared with different ratios of Pectin.

Formula	Drug content (%)		Standard deviation	Coefficient of variation %
	mean	range		
8tA	100.5	98-105	2.8	2.8
8tB	100.8	99-103	1.4	1.4
8tC	99.2	97-102	1.9	1.9
8tD	97.0	95-99	1.4	1.4
8tG	98.5	95-101	2.6	2.6

Table (51): Hardness values of metronidazole tablets prepared with different ratios of Pectin.

Formula	Hardness (Kg)		Standard deviation	Coefficient of variation %
	mean	range		
8tA	9.4	8-11	1.1	11.7
8tB	4.1	3-5	0.89	21.7
8tC	5.0	4-6	0.8	16
8tD	6.3	5-8	1.1	17.4
8tG	3.65	2.9-5	0.8	21.9

8; Polymer Pectin   t; tablet dosage form.

A; drug: polymer ratio 2:1   B; drug: polymer ratio 1:1

C; drug: polymer ratio 2:3   D; drug: polymer ratio 1:2

G; drug: polymer ratio 1:3

Table (52): Friability values of metronidazole tablets prepared with different ratios of Pectin.

Formula	Friability (%w/w)		Standard deviation	Coefficient of variation %
	mean	range		
8tA	0.195	0.18-0.21	0.01	5.1
8tB	0.85	0.8-0.9	0.04	4.7
8tC	0.7	0.68-0.8	0.05	7.1
8tD	0.9	0.8-1	0.08	8.9
8tG	1.026	0.96-1.2	0.09	8.8

Table (53): Disintegration times of metronidazole tablets prepared with different ratios of Pectin.

Formula	Disintegration time (min)		Standard deviation	Coefficient of variation %
	mean	range		
8tA	22	20-25	2.2	10
8tB	10.2	9-11	0.8	7.9
8tC	Tablets swell only			
8tD	Tablets swell only			
8tG	Tablets swell only			

8; Polymer Pectin   t; tablet dosage form.

A; drug: polymer ratio 2:1   B; drug: polymer ratio 1:1

C; drug: polymer ratio 2:3   D; drug: polymer ratio 1:2

G; drug: polymer ratio 1:3

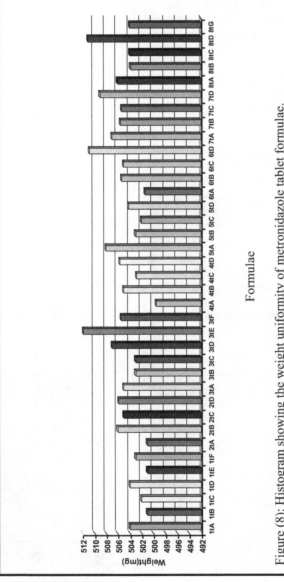

Figure (8): Histogram showing the weight uniformity of metronidazole tablet formulae.

A; drug: polymer ratio 2:1   B; drug: polymer ratio 1:1   C; drug: polymer ratio 2:3
D; drug: polymer ratio 1:2   E; drug: polymer ratio 4:1   F; drug: polymer ratio 3:1   G; drug: polymer ratio 1:3

1; HPMC 15000   2; HPMC 4000   3; Carbopol 934   4; Na alginate
5; CMC   6; Ethyl cellulose   7; Methyl cellulose   8; Pectin

122

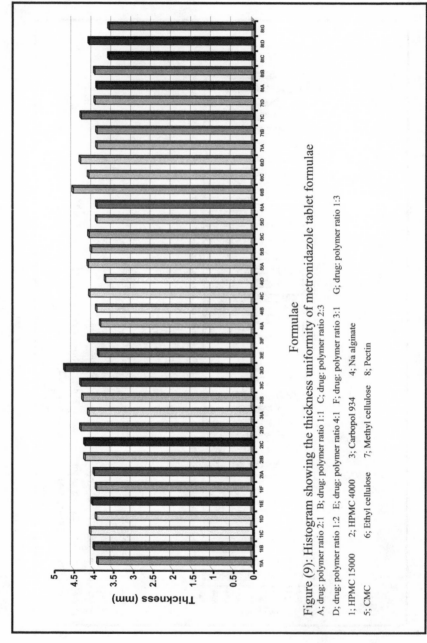

Formulae

Figure (9): Histogram showing the thickness uniformity of metronidazole tablet formulae

A; drug: polymer ratio 2:1   B; drug: polymer ratio 1:1   C; drug: polymer ratio 2:3

D; drug: polymer ratio 1:2   E; drug: polymer ratio 4:1   F; drug: polymer ratio 3:1   G; drug: polymer ratio 1:3

1; HPMC 15000   2; HPMC 4000   3; Carbopol 934   4; Na alginate

5; CMC   6; Ethyl cellulose   7; Methyl cellulose   8; Pectin

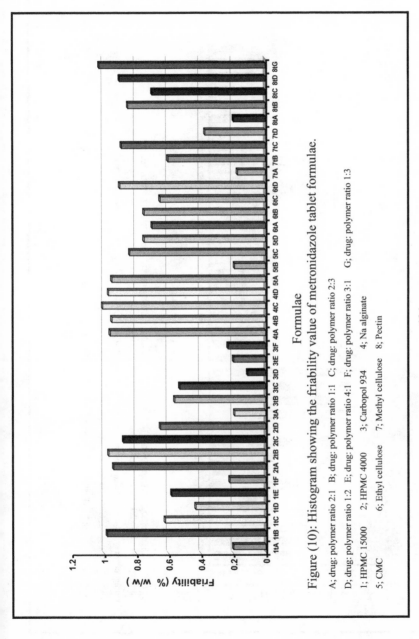

Figure (10): Histogram showing the friability value of metronidazole tablet formulae.

A; drug: polymer ratio 2:1 B; drug: polymer ratio 1:1 C; drug: polymer ratio 2:3
D; drug: polymer ratio 1:2 E; drug: polymer ratio 4:1 F; drug: polymer ratio 3:1 G; drug: polymer ratio 1:3

1; HPMC 15000   2; HPMC 4000   3; Carbopol 934   4; Na alginate
5; CMC   6; Ethyl cellulose   7; Methyl cellulose   8; Pectin

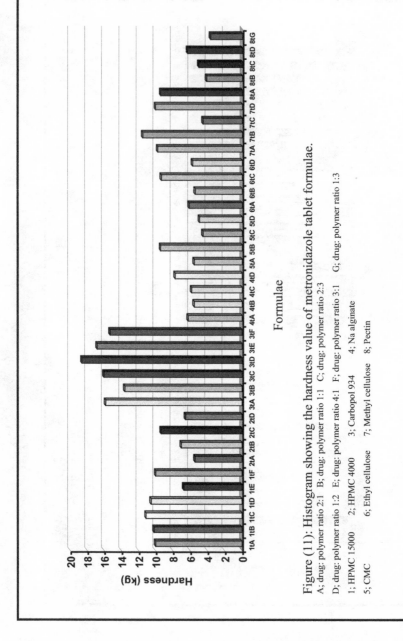

Figure (11): Histogram showing the hardness value of metronidazole tablet formulae.

A; drug: polymer ratio 2:1   B; drug: polymer ratio 1:1   C; drug: polymer ratio 2:3

D; drug: polymer ratio 1:2   E; drug: polymer ratio 4:1   F; drug: polymer ratio 3:1   G; drug: polymer ratio 1:3

1; HPMC 15000   2; HPMC 4000   3; Carbopol 934   4; Na alginate

5; CMC   6; Ethyl cellulose   7; Methyl cellulose   8; Pectin

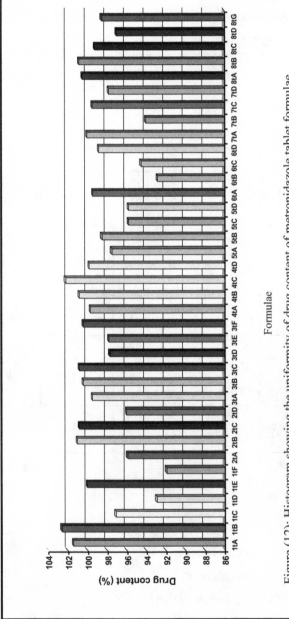

Formulae

Figure (12): Histogram showing the uniformity of drug content of metronidazole tablet formulae.

A; drug: polymer ratio 2:1   B; drug: polymer ratio 1:1   C; drug: polymer ratio 2:3

D; drug: polymer ratio 1:2   E; drug: polymer ratio 4:1   F; drug: polymer ratio 3:1   G; drug: polymer ratio 1:3

1; HPMC 15000   2; HPMC 4000   3; Carbopol 934   4; Na alginate

5; CMC   6; Ethyl cellulose   7; Methyl cellulose   8; Pectin

Table (54): The in-vitro release of metronidazole from its tablets containing HPMC 15000 with different drug: polymer ratios.

Dissolution medium	Time (hour)	% metronidazole released from						
		Plain tablet	1tA	1tB	1tC	1tD	1tE	1tF
0.1 N HCl pH 1.2	0	0	0	0	0	0	0	0
	0.5	81	18.7	18.34	21.6	14.9	62.6	74.7
	1.0	100	20.3	25.2	25.7	21.8	65.95	82.9
	1.5		28.7	35	28.4	32.2	78.2	86.6
	2.0		35.7	41.2	30	34.6	89.16	90.5
	2.5		38.6	46.4	38	36.6	93.07	95.4
	3.0		41.4	51.1	39	37.6	96.58	100
	3.5		57	53.7	42	43.6	100	
	4.0		62.4	56.6	53	48.2		
	4.5		67.5	57.2	54	51.1		
	5.0		70	57.7	56.5	55.4		
	5.5		71.2	63.8	58.3	58.7		
	6.0		73	66.5	64.2	59.5		

Plain tablet: the same ingredient without polymer.

1; HPMC 15000

t; tablet dosage form

A; drug: polymer ratio 2:1   B; drug: polymer ratio 1:1

C; drug: polymer ratio 2:3   D; drug: polymer ratio 1:2

E; drug: polymer ratio 3:1   F; drug: polymer ratio 4:1

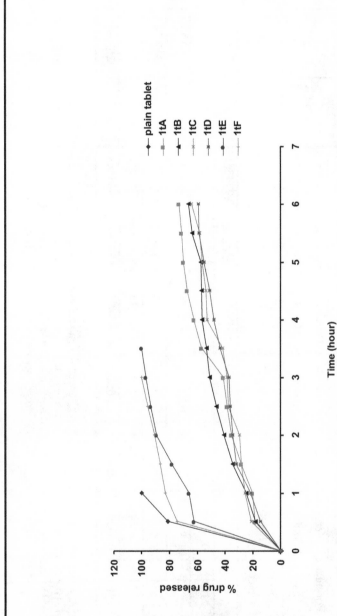

Figure (13): Release profiles of metronidazole from its tablet prepared with different ratio of HPMC 15000, into buffer solution of pH 1.2.

Table (55): Kinetics of the dissolution data of metronidazole from its tablets prepared with different ratios of HPMC 15000 polymer.

Formula	Correlation Coefficient (r)						*Rate constant K	t ½ (min)
	Zero-order	First-order	Second-order	Diffusion Model	Hixon-Crowl	Baker & Lonsdale		
Plain tablet	0.866025	-0.86603	0.866025	0.90143	0.866025	0.866025	4.89	104.45
1tA	0.981156	-0.98338	0.974279	0.978185	0.983981	0.974561	0.0045	208.64
1tB	0.960455	-0.98307	0.988143	0.988644	0.977295	0.99003	0.000305	180.06
1tC	0.98968	-0.98469	0.970478	0.975775	0.987339	0.972332	0.13137	380.75
1tD	0.983104	-0.9915	0.987362	0.991418	0.990164	0.986763	0.00222	312.78
1tE	0.972017	-0.88259	0.629912	0.981815	0.976576	0.987817	0.0022	25.004
1tF	0.991994	-0.83739	0.665219	0.995879	0.937543	0.965543	3.05	268.65

*K value (dissolution rate constant) & t ½ were calculated according to the order of drug release.

1; HPMC 15000

A; Drug: polymer ratio 2:1
D; drug: polymer ratio 1:2

t; tablet dosage form
B; drug: polymer ratio 1:1
E; drug: polymer ratio 3:1

plain tablet; the same ingredient without polymer
C; drug: polymer ratio 2:3
F; drug: polymer ratio 4:1

129

Table (56): In-vitro release of metronidazole from its tablets containing HPMC 4000 in different drug: polymer ratios.

Dissolution medium	Time (hour)	% metronidazole released from				
		Plain tablet	2tA	2tB	2tC	2tD
0.1 N HCl pH 1.2	0	0	0	0	0	0
	0.5	81	73	41.7	38.6	28
	1.0	100	81.8	58.6	46.4	39.5
	1.5		86.6	63.4	55.6	46.8
	2.0		88.5	67.9	62.1	53.4
	2.5		88.95	72.6	68.2	56.3
	3.0		89.6	80.6	76.3	60.9
	3.5		95.88	85.9	78.9	68.6
	4.0		99.5	92.9	85.2	76.9
	4.5			94.5	87.5	77.8
	5.0			98.9	90.9	84.9
	5.5			100	91.9	85.5
	6.0				92	91.7

Plain tablet: the same ingredient without polymer.

2; HPMC 4000

t; tablet dosage form

A; drug: polymer ratio 2:1   B; drug: polymer ratio 1:1

C; drug: polymer ratio 2:3   D; drug: polymer ratio 1:2

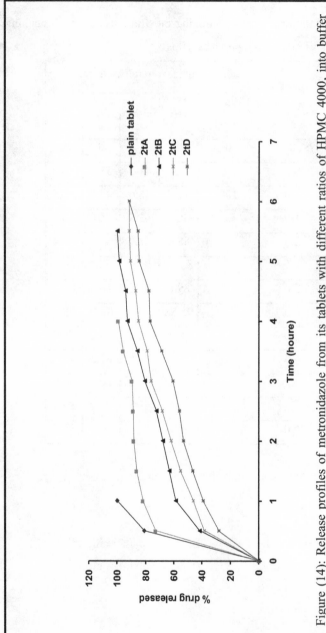

Figure (14): Release profiles of metronidazole from its tablets with different ratios of HPMC 4000, into buffer solution of pH 1.2.

131

Table (57): Kinetics of the dissolution data of metronidazole from its tablets prepared with different ratios of HPMC 4000 polymer.

Formula	Correlation Coefficient (r)							*Rate constant K	t ½ (min)
	Zero-order	First-order	Second-order	Diffusion-Model	Hixon-Crowel	Baker& Lonsdale			
Plain tablet	0.866025	-0.86603	0.866025	0.90143	0.866025	0.866025	4.89	104.45
2tA	0.950958	-0.84661	0.636643	0.965905	0.919706	0.936202	2.283	479.48
2tB	0.97864	-0.88183	0.547837	0.993449	0.974914	0.978539	4.56	120.05
2tC	0.969031	-0.99412	0.959339	0.992237	0.992808	0.992857	0.0068	101.66
2tD	0.989524	-0.97814	0.87734	0.995461	0.991672	0.978375	4.66	114.9

*K value (dissolution rate constant) & t ½ were calculated according to the order of drug release.

plain tablet; the same ingredient without polymer

2; HPMC 4000   t; tablet dosage form

A; Drug: polymer ratio 2:1   B; drug: polymer ratio 1:1

C; drug: polymer ratio 2:3   D; drug: polymer ratio 1:2

Table (58): In-vitro release of metronidazole from its tablets containing Carbopol 934 in different drug: polymer ratios.

Dissolution medium	Time (hour)	% metronidazole released from						
		Plain tablet	3tA	3tB	3tC	3tD	3tE	3tF
0.1 N HCl pH 1.2	0	0	0	0	0	0	0	0
	0.5	81	16.8	27.7	26.3	34.1	30.82	57.17
	1.0	100	21.9	34	35	37.5	41.95	75.9
	1.5		31.8	38.6	41.4	43.4	53.65	93.85
	2.0		38	44	44.1	44.4	63.21	95.02
	2.5		43.5	49.5	49.3	45.4	70	100
	3.0		50.3	55.6	55	51.7	78	
	3.5		66.5	60.2	57.1	53.7	85.07	
	4.0		70	63.1	60.8	60	95.1	
	4.5		73.8	65.9	63.6	63.4	100	
	5.0		79	69.9	67.7	65.8		
	5.5		81.9	72	70	69.3		
	6.0		85.1	74	73.9	73.2		

Plain tablet: the same ingredient without polymer.

3; Carbopol 934

t; tablet dosage form

A; drug: polymer ratio 2:1   B; drug: polymer ratio 1:1

C; drug: polymer ratio 2:3   D; drug: polymer ratio 1:2

E; drug: polymer ratio 3:1   F; drug: polymer ratio 4:1

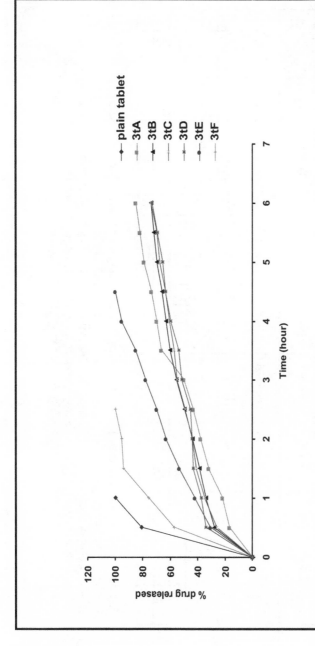

Figure (15): Release profiles of metronidazole from its tablets with different ratios of Carbopol 934, into buffer solution of pH 1.2.

Table (59): Kinetics of the dissolution data of metronidazole from its tablets prepared with different ratios of Carbopol 934 polymer.

Formula	Correlation Coefficient (r)						*Rate constant K	t ½ (min)
	Zero-order	First-order	Second-order	Diffusion-Model	Hixon-Crowl	Baker& Lonsdale		
Plain tablet	0.866025	-0.86603	0.866025	0.90143	0.866025	0.866025	4.89	104.45
3tA	0.98711	-0.98996	0.95282	0.988355	0.993105	0.979967	0.0061	155.78
3tB	0.988201	-0.99862	0.991643	0.996907	0.997024	0.996937	0.0032	216.27
3tC	0.988413	-0.99773	0.984007	0.998636	0.99716	0.995218	3.44	210.66
3tD	0.994986	-0.98685	0.964726	0.980117	0.991114	0.979559	0.11817	423.11
3tE	0.995408	-0.81416	0.559019	0.997607	0.945144	0.940794	6.403	60.96
3tF	0.933135	-0.91445	0.718677	0.96492	0.979595	0.981621	0.0033	16.39

*K value (dissolution rate constant) & t ½ were calculated according to the order of drug release.
plain tablet; the same ingredient without polymer

A; Drug: polymer ratio 2:1   B; drug: polymer ratio 1:1   C; drug: polymer ratio 2:3
D; drug: polymer ratio 1:2   E; drug: polymer ratio 3:1   F; drug: polymer ratio 4:1
3; Carbopol 934   t; tablet dosage form

135

Table (60): In-vitro release of metronidazole from its tablets containing Na alginate in different drug: polymer ratios.

Dissolution medium	Time (hour)	% metronidazole released from				
		Plain tablet	4tA	4tB	4tC	4tD
0.1 N HCl pH 1.2	0	0	0	0	0	0
	0.5	81	81	42.9	29.3	34.5
	1.0	100	83.3	44.7	40.6	51
	1.5		86.4	48.6	43.9	85.3
	2.0		87.2	58.7	52.1	100
	2.5		89.4	70.2	56.2	
	3.0		90	73.7	58.5	
	3.5		94.4	77.1	66	
	4.0		100	79	66.3	
	4.5			88.9	66.5	
	5.0			79.4	72.7	
	5.5			100	73.2	
	6.0				78	

Plain tablet: the same ingredient without polymer.

4; Na alginate

t; tablet dosage form

A; drug: polymer ratio 2:1   B; drug: polymer ratio 1:1

C; drug: polymer ratio 2:3   D; drug: polymer ratio 1:2

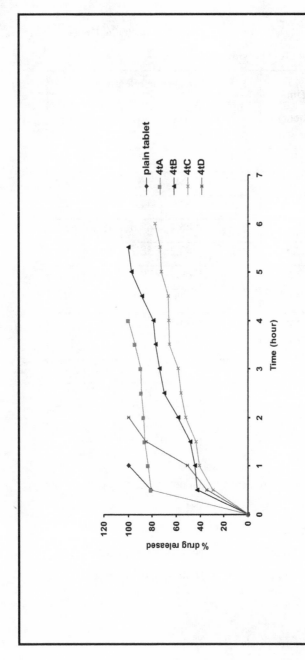

Figure (16): Release profiles of metronidazole from its tablets with different ratios of Na alginate, into buffer solution of pH 1.2.

137

Table (61): Kinetics of the dissolution data of metronidazole from its tablets prepared with different ratios of Na alginate polymer.

Formula	Correlation Coefficient (r)						*Rate constant K	t ½ (min)
	Zero-order	First-order	Second-order	Diffusion-Model	Hixon-Crowl	Baker& Lonsdale		
Plain tablet	0.866025	-0.86603	0.866025	0.90143	0.866025	0.866025	4.89	104.45
4tA	0.969011	-0.73049	0.585286	0.944724	0.837157	0.879005	0.0796	627.49
4tB	0.989507	-0.80441	0.519875	0.97889	0.928914	0.927838	0.20127	248.419
4tC	0.971099	-0.9896	0.978052	0.992267	0.986615	0.990516	3.43	211.898
4tD	0.98686	-0.88451	0.777322	0.98155	0.957026	0.952039	0.7683	65.0759

* K value (dissolution rate constant) & t ½ were calculated according to the order of drug release.
plain tablet; the same ingredient without polymer
A; Drug: polymer ratio 2:1   B; drug: polymer ratio 1:1
C; drug: polymer ratio 2:3   D; drug: polymer ratio 1:2
4; Na alginate   t; tablet dosage form

138

Table (62): In-vitro release of metronidazole from its tablets containing CMC in different drug: polymer ratios.

Dissolution medium	Time (hour)	% metronidazole released from				
		Plain tablet	5tA	5tB	5tC	5tD
0.1 N HCl pH 1.2	0	0	0	0	0	0
	0.5	81	56.7	42.9	27.3	21.6
	1.0	100	64.4	49.4	37.5	24.4
	1.5		69.1	64.4	44.9	36.7
	2.0		77.8	69.6	49.7	43.3
	2.5		81.4	71.2	58.7	51.7
	3.0		82.5	72.9	63.8	58.3
	3.5		84.1	76.2	76.9	61.7
	4.0		88	80	79.6	69.1
	4.5		92.1	82.1	85.1	72.9
	5.0		97.8	87	85.1	74.3
	5.5		100	79.2	88.2	74.3
	6.0			99.5	100	77.6

Plain tablet: the same ingredient without polymer.

5; CMC

t; tablet dosage form

A; drug: polymer ratio 2:1   B; drug: polymer ratio 1:1

C; drug: polymer ratio 2:3   D; drug: polymer ratio 1:2

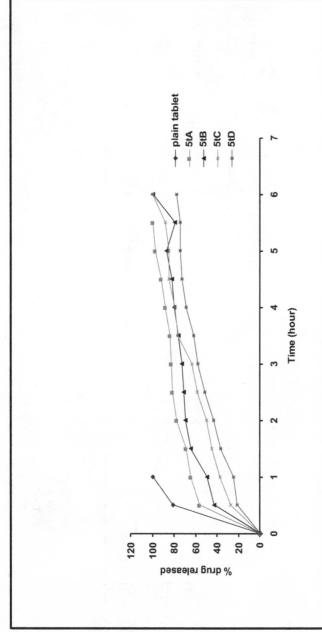

Figure (17): Release profiles of metronidazole from its tablets with different ratios of CMC, into buffer solution of pH 1.2.

Table (63): Kinetics of the dissolution data of metronidazole from its tablets prepared with different ratios of CMC polymer.

Formula	Correlation Coefficient (r)						*Rate constant K	t ½ (min)
	Zero-order	First-order	Second-order	Diffusion-Model	Hixon-Crowl	Baker&Lonsdale		
Plain tablet	0.866025	-0.86603	0.866025	0.90143	0.866025	0.866025	4.89	104.45
5tA	0.981567	-0.81531	0,524217	0.991868	0.938214	0.954849	3.295	230.17
5tB	0.970052	-0.83453	0.565386	0.97938	0.924053	0.920341	3.878	166.23
5tC	0.986292	-0.75234	0.48724	0.991392	0.920642	0.917933	5.3005	88.98
5tD	0.969769	-0.99053	0.988418	0.989047	0.986112	0.990292	0.00407	170.257

* K value (dissolution rate constant) & t ½ were calculated according to the order of drug release.
plain tablet; the same ingredient without polymer

A; Drug: polymer ratio 2:1   B; drug: polymer ratio 1:1

C; drug: polymer ratio 2:3   D; drug: polymer ratio 1:2

5; CMC   t; tablet dosage form

141

Table (64): In-vitro release of metronidazole from its tablets containing ethyl cellulose in different drug: polymer ratios.

Dissolution medium	Time (hour)	% metronidazole released from				
		Plain tablet	6tA	6tB	6tC	6tD
0.1 N HCl pH 1.2	0	0	0	0	0	0
	0.5	81	97.4	92.2	92	90
	1.0	100	99.9	94.5	94	92
	1.5			96.7	96.3	97.2
	2.0			100	100	100
	2.5					
	3.0					
	3.5					
	4.0					
	4.5					
	5.0					
	5.5					
	6.0					

Plain tablet: the same ingredient without polymer.

6; ethyl cellulose

t; tablet dosage form

A; drug: polymer ratio 2:1   B; drug: polymer ratio 1:1
C; drug: polymer ratio 2:3   D; drug: polymer ratio 1:2

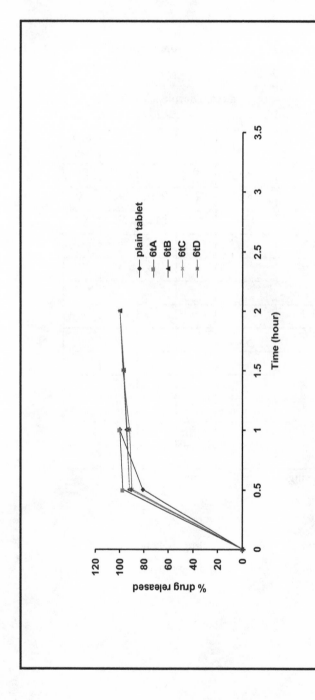

Figure (18): Release profiles of metronidazole from its tablets with different ratios of Ethyl cellulose, into buffer solution of pH 1.2.

Table (65): Kinetics of the dissolution data of metronidazole from its tablets prepared with different ratios of Ethyl cellulose polymer.

Formula	Correlation Coefficient (r)							*Rate constant K	t ½ (min)
	Zero-order	First-order	Second-order	Diffusion-Model	Hixon-Crowl	Baker& Lonsdale			
Plain tablet	0.866025	-0.86603	0.866025	0.90143	0.866025	0.866025	4.89	104.45
6tA	0.86605	-0.86603	0.866025	0.90143	0.86625	0.866025	0.647	5949.8
6tB	0.995916	-0.87312	0.783726	0.983849	0.928626	0.958288	0.084	592.88
6tC	0.989947	-0.86273	0.782181	0.972245	0.915878	0.945487	0.0866	576.9
6tD	0.985958	-0.90229	0.787919	0.974525	0.954426	0.973081	0.1163	429.79

* K value (dissolution rate constant) & t ½ were calculated according to the order of drug release.
plain tablet; the same ingredient without polymer

A; Drug: polymer ratio 2:1   B; drug: polymer ratio 1:1
C; drug: polymer ratio 2:3   D; drug: polymer ratio 1:2
6; Ethyl cellulose   t; tablet dosage form

144

Table (66): In-vitro release of metronidazole from its tablets containing methyl cellulose in different drug: polymer ratios.

Dissolution medium	Time (hour)	% metronidazole released from				
		Plain tablet	7tA	7tB	7tC	7tD
0.1 N HCl pH 1.2	0	0	0	0	0	0
	0.5	81	24.2	30.6	29.2	20.1
	1.0	100	31.4	33.9	33.6	33.5
	1.5		40.6	51	42.9	45.8
	2.0		51.3	55.4	49.2	49.7
	2.5		53.3	60.4	56.6	60
	3.0		62	72.6	64.6	63.8
	3.5		76.7	73.5	65	64.7
	4.0		81.2	78.8	72.8	71.2
	4.5		84.7	82.7	74	73.1
	5.0		86.6	84.1	76	74.5
	5.5		88.8	87.9	79	79.2
	6.0		93.1	89.7	84	83.7

Plain tablet: the same ingredient without polymer.

7; methyl cellulose

t; tablet dosage form

A; drug: polymer ratio 2:1   B; drug: polymer ratio 1:1

C; drug: polymer ratio 2:3   D; drug: polymer ratio 1:2

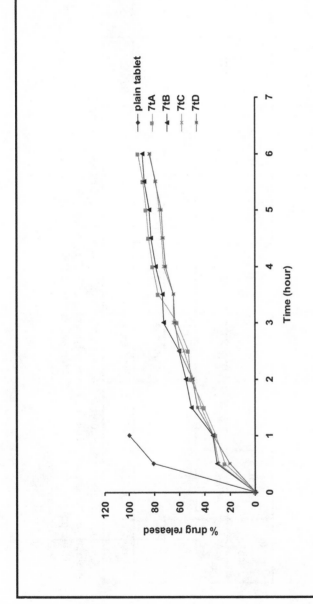

Figure (19): Release profiles of metronidazole from its tablets with different ratios of Methyl cellulose, into buffer solution of pH 1.2.

Table (67): Kinetics of the dissolution data of metronidazole from its tablets prepared with different ratios of Methyl cellulose polymer.

Formula	Correlation Coefficient (r)						*Rate constant K	t ½ (min)
	Zero-order	First-order	Second-order	Diffusion-Model	Hixon-Crowl	Baker&Lonsdale		
Plain tablet	0.866025	-0.86603	0.866025	0.90143	0.866025	0.866025	4.89	104.45
7tA	0.978531	-0.98715	0.90748	0.98924	0.991982	0.983975	0.00724	131.933
7tB	0.966431	-0.99578	0.959761	0.988416	0.992661	0.994876	0.00592	117.05
7tC	0.978547	-0.99392	0.964793	0.993377	0.993067	0.992515	0.00438	158.319
7tD	0.958328	-0.99101	0.963657	0.988706	0.986135	0.992864	0.00059	93.139

* K value (dissolution rate constant) & t ½ were calculated according to the order of drug release.
plain tablet; the same ingredient without polymer

A; Drug: polymer ratio 2:1   B; drug: polymer ratio 1:1
C; drug: polymer ratio 2:3   D; drug: polymer ratio 1:2
7; Methyl cellulose   t; tablet dosage form

147

Table (68): In-vitro release of metronidazole from its tablets containing pectin in different drug: polymer ratios.

Dissolution medium	Time (hour)	% metronidazole released from					
		Plain tablet	8tA	8tB	8tC	8tD	8tG
0.1 N HCl pH 1.2	0	0	0	0	0	0	0
	0.5	81	77.5	77	76.5	30	22.4
	1.0	100	100	100	90.1	35.9	28.8
	1.5				100	44.8	38.4
	2.0					45.5	42.1
	2.5					55	50.1
	3.0					61.8	59.9
	3.5					66.5	66.3
	4.0					72.4	67.3
	4.5					79	77.4
	5.0					80	73.9
	5.5					81.2	76.3
	6.0					86.2	76.3

Plain tablet: same ingredient without polymer.

8; pectin

t; tablet dosage form

A; drug: polymer ratio 2:1   B; drug: polymer ratio 1:1

C; drug: polymer ratio 2:3   D; drug: polymer ratio 1:2

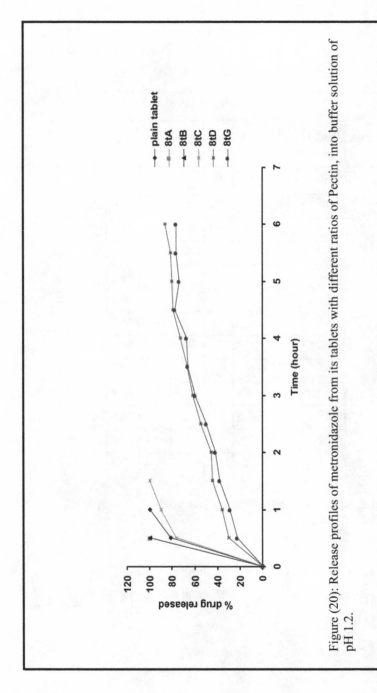

Figure (20): Release profiles of metronidazole from its tablets with different ratios of Pectin, into buffer solution of pH 1.2.

Table (69): Kinetics of the dissolution data of metronidazole from its tablets prepared with different ratios of Pectin polymer.

Formula	Correlation Coefficient (r)						*Rate constant K	t½ (min)
	Zero-order	First-order	Second-order	Diffusion-Model	Hixon-Crowl	Baker&Lonsdale		
Plain tablet	0.866025	-0.86603	0.866025	0.90143	0.866025	0.866025	4.89	104.45
8tA	0.982292	-0.89767	0.866991	0.971906	0.927626	0.937533	0.746667	66.964
8tB	0.950969	0.88529	0.86655	0.934633	0.9053430	0.911551	0.7633	65.50
8tC	0.995634	-0.93023	0.868564	0.999845	0.97405	0.98617	5.8438	73.206
8tD	0.98759	-0.99127	0.953445	0.99198	0.994357	0.987518	0.005315	122.28
8tG	0.963802	-0.97464	0.963286	0.983453	0.973516	0.971912	4.52	122.28

* K value (dissolution rate constant) & t ½ were calculated according to the order of drug release.

plain tablet; the same ingredient without polymer

A; Drug: polymer ratio 2:1   B; drug: polymer ratio 1:1
C; drug: polymer ratio 2:3   D; drug: polymer ratio 1:2   G; drug: polymer ratio 1:3
8; Pectin   t; tablet dosage form

150

Table (70): In-vitro release of metronidazole from tablets using different polymers with drug: polymer ratio 2:1.

Dissolution medium	Time (hour)	% metronidazole released from							
		1tA	2tA	3tA	4tA	5tA	6tA	7tA	8tA
0.1 N HCl pH 1.2	0	0	0	0	0	0	0	0	0
	0.5	18.7	73	16.8	81	56.7	97.4	24.2	77.5
	1.0	20.3	81.8	21.9	83.3	64.4	99.9	31.4	100
	1.5	28.7	86.6	31.8	86.4	69.1		40.6	
	2.0	35.7	88.5	38	87.2	77.8		51.3	
	2.5	38.6	88.95	43.5	89.4	81.4		53.3	
	3.0	41.4	89.6	50.3	90	82.5		62	
	3.5	57	95.88	66.5	94.4	84.1		76.7	
	4.0	62.4	99.5	70	100	88		81.2	
	4.5	67.5		73.8		92.1		84.7	
	5.0	70		79		97.8		86.6	
	5.5	71.2		81.9		100		88.8	
	6.0	73		85.1				93.1	

A; drug: polymer ratio 2:1

t; tablet dosage form

1; HPMC 15000   2; HPMC 4000   3; Carbopol 934   4; Na alginate

5; CMC   6; Ethyl cellulose   7; Methyl cellulose   8; Pectin

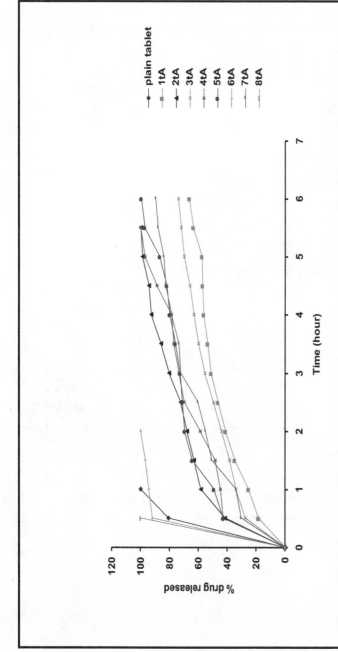

Figure (21): Release profiles of metronidazole from its tablets prepared with different polymers using drug: polymer ratio 2:1, into buffer solution of pH 1.2.

Table (71): In-vitro release of metronidazole from tablets using different polymers with drug: polymer ratio 1:1.

Dissolution medium	Time (hour)	% metronidazole released from							
		1tB	2tB	3tB	4tB	5tB	6tB	7tB	8tB
0.1 N HCl pH 1.2	0	0	0	0	0	0	0	0	0
	0.5	18.34	41.7	27.7	42.9	42.9	92.2	30.6	77
	1.0	25.2	58.6	34	44.7	49.4	94.5	33.9	100
	1.5	35	63.4	38.6	48.6	64.4	96.7	51	
	2.0	41.2	67.9	44	58.7	69.6	100	55.4	
	2.5	46.2	72.6	49.5	70.2	71.2		60.4	
	3.0	51.1	80.6	55.6	73.7	72.9		72.6	
	3.5	53.7	85.9	60.2	77.1	76.2		73.5	
	4.0	56.6	92.9	63.1	79	80		78.8	
	4.5	57.2	94.5	65.9	88.9	82.1		82.7	
	5.0	57.7	98.9	69.9	97.4	87		84.1	
	5.5	63.8	100	72	100	97.2		87.9	
	6.0	66.5		74		99.5		89.7	

B; drug: polymer ratio 1:1

t; tablet dosage form

1; HPMC 15000   2; HPMC 4000   3; Carbopol 934   4; Na alginate

5; CMC   6; Ethyl cellulose   7; Methyl cellulose   8; Pectin

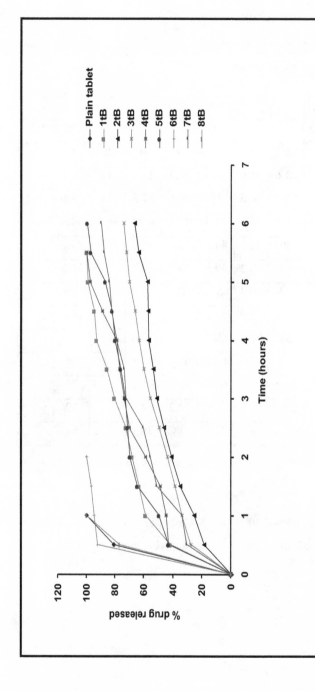

Figure (22): Release profiles of metronidazole from its tablets prepared with different polymers using drug: polymer ratio 1:1, into buffer solution of pH 1.2.

Table (72): In-vitro release of metronidazole from tablets using different polymers with drug: polymer ratio 2:3.

Dissolution medium	Time (hour)	% metronidazole released from							
		1tC	2tC	3tC	4tC	5tC	6tC	7tC	8tC
0.1 N HCl pH 1.2	0	0	0	0	0	0	0	0	0
	0.5	21.6	38.6	26.3	29.3	27.3	92	29.2	76.5
	1.0	25.7	46.6	35	40.6	37.5	94	33.6	90.1
	1.5	28.4	55.6	41.4	43.9	44.9	96.3	42.9	100
	2.0	30	62.1	44.1	52.1	49.9	100	49.2	
	2.5	38	68.2	49.3	56.2	58.7		56.6	
	3.0	39	76.3	55	58.5	63.8		64.6	
	3.5	42	78.9	57.1	66	76.9		65	
	4.0	53	85.2	60.8	66.3	79.6		72.8	
	4.5	54	87.5	63.6	66.5	85.1		74	
	5.0	56.5	90.9	67.7	72.7	85.1		76	
	5.5	58.3	91.9	70	73.2	88.2		79	
	6.0	64.2	92	73.9	78	100		84	

C; drug: polymer ratio 2:3

t; tablet dosage form

1; HPMC 15000   2; HPMC 4000   3; Carbopol 934   4; Na alginate

5; CMC   6; Ethyl cellulose   7; Methyl cellulose   8; Pectin

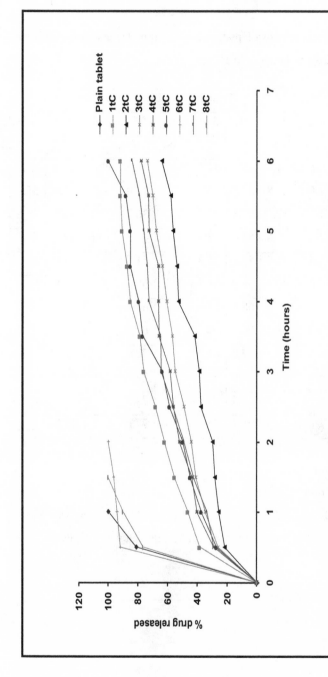

Figure (23): Release profiles of metronidazole from its tablets prepared with different polymers using drug: polymer ratio 2:3, into buffer solution of pH 1.2.

Table (73): In-vitro release of metronidazole from tablets using different polymers with drug: polymer ratio 1:2.

Dissolution medium	Time (hour)	% metronidazole released from							
		1tD	2tD	3tD	4tD	5tD	6tD	7tD	8tD
0.1 N HCl pH 1.2	0	0	0	0	0	0	0	0	0
	0.5	14.9	28	34.1	34.5	21.6	90	20.1	30
	1.0	21.8	39.5	37.5	51	24.4	92	33.9	35.9
	1.5	32.2	46.8	43.4	85.3	36.7	97.2	45.8	44.8
	2.0	34.6	53.4	44.4	100	43.3	100	49.7	45.5
	2.5	36.6	56.3	45.4		51.7		60	55
	3.0	37.6	60.9	51.7		58.3		63.8	61.8
	3.5	43.6	68.6	53.7		61.7		64.7	66.5
	4.0	48.2	76.9	60		69.1		71.2	72.4
	4.5	51.1	77.8	63.4		72.9		73.12	79
	5.0	55.4	84.9	65.8		74.3		74.5	80
	5.5	58.7	85.5	69.3		74.3		79.2	81.2
	6.0	59.5	91.7	73.2		77.6		83.7	86.2

D; drug: polymer ratio 1:2

t; tablet dosage form

1; HPMC 15000   2; HPMC 4000   3; Carbopol 934   4; Na alginate

5; CMC   6; Ethyl cellulose   7; Methyl cellulose   8; Pectin

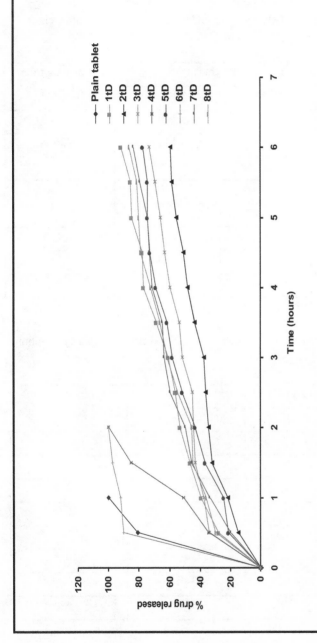

Figure (24): Release profiles of metronidazole from its tablets prepared with different polymers using drug: polymer ratio 1:2, into buffer solution of pH 1.2.

Table (74): The relation between metronidazole tablet lag time and weight of gas generating layer.

Gas generating layer weight (mg)			Tablet lag time
$CaCO_3$	$NaHCO_3$	HPMC 4000	(minutes)
5	2.5	140	60
10	5	140	25
15	7.5	140	7
20	10	140	5
25	12.5	140	4
30	15	140	4
35	17.5	140	4
40	20	140	3

*Gas generating mixture $CaCO_3$:$NaHCO_3$ used in ratio (2:1).

Table (75): The relation between metronidazole tablet buoyancy duration and weight of gas generating layer.

Gas generating layer weight (mg)			Buoyancy duration
$CaCO_3$	$NaHCO_3$	HPMC 4000	(hours)
5	2.5	140	6
10	5	140	6
15	7.5	140	6
20	10	140	6
25	12.5	140	6
30	15	140	6
35	17.5	140	6
40	20	140	6

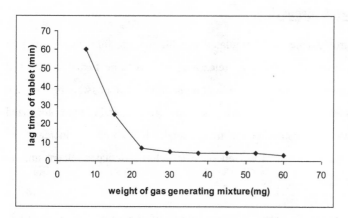

Figure (25): The relation between metronidazole tablet lag time and weight of gas generating mixture (CaCO$_3$: NaHCO$_3$ 2:1).

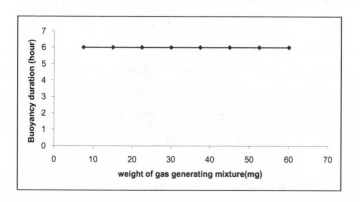

Figure (26): The relation between metronidazole tablet buoyancy duration and weight of gas generating mixture (CaCO$_3$: NaHCO$_3$ 2:1).

Results and Discussion

Metronidazole was formulated in tablet dosage form using different polymers in order to retard the release as well as to be floatable over 6-8 hours on the gastric content. The floating features could possibly prolong the gastric retention time of those systems to maintain high localized concentration of metronidazole in the stomach in order to increase the efficacy of the therapy for Helicobacter pylori associated ulcers and to improve patient compliance.

Metronidazole exhibited a maximum absorbance at 278 nm in 0.1 N HCl medium when measured spectrophotometrically. Table (4) and Figure (7) showed the standard calibration curve of metronidazole in 0.1 N HCl. A linear curve was produced between the concentrations of metronidazole and its absorbance which obeys Beer's Lambert law. The value of correlation coefficient was 0.9992.

Tables (6, 12, 18, 24, 30, 36, 42, and 48) showed the uniformity of weight of metronidazole tablets manufactured by direct compression technique. It is clear from the tables that the weight of the tested tablets complied with the pharmaceutical compendia in B.P (1993).

The tablets showed coefficient of variation less than 3% which mean excellent uniformity of weight. Metronidazole tablets containing polymer methyl cellulose in drug: polymer ratio2:3 (formula 7tC) showed the lowest coefficient of variation of weight (0.06) while metronidazole tablets containing polymer HPMC 15000 with drug: polymer ratio 2:1 (formula 1tA) showed the highest coefficient of variation of weight (1.4). Figure (8)

161

showed a histogram illustrating the uniformity of weight of metronidazole tablet formulae.

The uniformity of thickness, in spite of being non official, can be considered as an additional control to the tablet dimension and increased reproducibility.

Tables (7, 13, 19, 25, 31, 37, 43, and 49), explained the thickness of metronidazole tablet formulae prepared by direct compression technique. The average thickness value of metronidazole tablets ranged from 3.6 mm to 4.7 mm with standard deviation ranges of 0.04 to 0.3. Metronidazole tablet prepared with polymer ethyl cellulose in drug: polymer ratio 1:2 (formula 6tD) showed the lowest coefficient of variation of thickness, while metronidazole tablet prepared with polymer pectin in drug: polymer ratio 2:3 (formula 8tC) showed the highest coefficient of variation of thickness.

These results indicate that all the prepared metronidazole tablet with different polymers in different drug: polymer ratios had acceptable limits of thickness uniformity. Figure (9) showed a histogram of thickness uniformity of metronidazole tablet formulae.

Tables (8, 14, 20, 26, 32, 38, 44, and 50) showed the uniformity of drug content of metronidazole tablets manufactured by direct compression technique. It is clear from the tables that the average drug content of metronidazole tablets ranged from 91.9% to 102.6 % with standard deviation ranged from 0.12 to 2.8. Metronidazole tablets prepared with polymer HPMC 4000 in drug: polymer ratio 2:1(formula 2tA) showed the lowest

162

coefficient of variation of drug content (0.12), while metronidazole tablets prepared with polymer methyl cellulose in drug: polymer ratio 2:1(formula 7tA) showed the highest coefficient of variation of drug content (13.1).All the investigated tablets complied with the pharmacopeal requirement for their drug content uniformity which found to lie between ±10%. Figure (10) showed a histogram of metronidazole tablet formulae and their drug content uniformity.

The mechanical properties of the investigated tablets were evaluated by testing their hardness and friability.

Tables (9, 15, 21, 27, 33, 39, 45, and 51) showed the hardness values of different metronidazole tablet formulae manufactured by direct compression technique. The average hardness values ranges from 3.65 kg to 18.6 kg with standard deviation values between 0.08 and 1.2. Metronidazole tablets containing polymer HPMC 15000 with drug: polymer ratio 4:1(formula 1tF) showed the lowest coefficient of variation of hardness (1%), while metronidazole tablets containing polymer methyl cellulose with drug: polymer ratio 2:3 (formula 7tC) showed the highest coefficient of variation of hardness (24.4%). Figure (11) showed a histogram of metronidazole tablet hardness values.

Tables (10, 16, 22, 28, 34, 40, 46, and 52) illustrate the results of the friability study of different metronidazole tablet formulae manufactured by direct compression technique. Average percent loss of weight ranges from 0.11 % to 1.026 %with standard deviation range from 0.002 to 0.1. Metronidazole tablets containing both polymers HPMC 4000 in drug:

163

polymer ratio 2:3 (formula 2tC) and polymer Carbopol 934 in drug: polymer ratio 2:1(3tA) showed the lowest coefficient of variation of percent loss of weight (1.1%).While metronidazole tablets containing polymer methyl cellulose in drug: polymer ratio 2:1 (7tA) showed the highest coefficient of variation of percent loss of weight (23.5%). Figure (12) showed a histogram of metronidazole tablet friability values.

According to USP 2000, complete disintegration is defined as that state in which any residue of the unit except fragment of insoluble coating or capsule shell, remaining on the screen of the test apparatus is a soft mass having no palably film core.

Tables (11, 17, 23, 29, 35, 41, 47, and 53) showed the disintegration time of different tablet formulae manufactured by direct compression. As shown in the tables, the values of disintegration time ranges from 2.75 to 34.3 minutes with standard deviation ranges from 0.8 to 4.1.Whereas tablets of metronidazole containing polymers HPMC 15000 in drug: polymer ratios 2:1, 1:1, 2:3, 1:2 (formulae 1tA, 1tB, 1tC, and 1tD) , polymer HPMC 4000 in drug: polymer ratios 2:1, 1:1, 2:3, and 1:2 (formulae 2tA, 2tB, 2tC, and 2tD, respectively) , polymer Carbopol 934 in drug: polymer ratios 2:1, 1:1, 2:3, and 1:2 (formulae 3tA, 3tB, 3tC, and 3tD, respectively),polymer sodium alginate in drug: polymer ratio 1:1 (formula 4tB), polymer CMC in drug: polymer ratios 2:1, 1:1, 2:3, and 1:2 (formula 5tA,5tB,5tC,and 5tD, respectively) , polymer methyl cellulose in drug: polymer ratio s 2:3, and 1:2 (formulae 7tC, and 7tD, respectively), and finally polymer pectin in drug: polymer ratios 2:3, 1:2, and 1:3 (formulae 8tC, 8tD, and 8tG, respectively) have no disintegration time as they only swell in the disintegration medium.

164

The previous tests gave an identification of good inter-batch uniformity for the prepared formulae of metronidazole tablets.

In-vitro release of metronidazole from conventional slow-release tablet dosage form

1-Formulae obtained using HPMC 15000

The contents of the metronidazole tablets containing different ratios of HPMC 15000 were given by Table (5a).

The dissolution rate of metronidazole from its conventional slow-release tablet formulae manufactured by direct compression technique containing different ratios of polymer HPMC 15000 are shown in Table (54), and illustrated in Figure (13). It is clear that, those formulae which contain drug: polymer ratios 3:1 and 4:1 showed rapid release of their drug content and reach maximum release of 100% within 3, and 3.5 hours respectively. In contrast, those formulae containing drug: polymer ratios 2:1 , 1:1, 2:3 and 1:2 showed slower release of their metronidazole content, and reach maximum release of (73%, 66.5%, 64.2%, and 59.5 respectively) after 6 hours dissolution.

It is clear that ,by increasing the ratio of HPMC 15000 in the prepared formulae (i.e. from drug: polymer ratio 4:1 to 3:1 then 2:1 then 1:1 then 2:3 and finally 1:2) the dissolution rates of the drug were slowed and the total percent released were decreased. These results were in accordance with the conclusion by Thanoo et al., (1993) and Suwannee et al., (1995) who concluded that, the increase in HPMC content caused a decrease in the percent of drug release. This could be explained by the swelling of HPMC after absorbing water, where a higher amount of HPMC absorbed more water and caused a greater degree of swelling. This in turn increased the tortousity and the length of the drug diffusional path, hence, decreasing the amount of drug released.

In order to explore the mechanism of drug release from these formulae the experimental dissolution data were tried on the basis of zero, first, second order as well as Diffusion controlled model (Higuchi, 1963), Hixson-Crowell Cube root law (Hixson and Crowell, 1977) and Baker and Lonsdale equation (Baker and Lonsdale, 1974) at pH 1.2.

It can be observed from Table (55) that the order of release for metronidazole from its tablets containing HPMC 15000 with drug: polymer ratio 1:1 (formula 1tB) and drug: polymer ratio 3:1 (formula 1tE) were found to obey Baker and Lonsdale equation with $t_{1/2}$ of 180.06, and 25.004 minutes respectively. While metronidazole tablets containing HPMC 15000 in drug: polymer ratio4:1 (formula 1tF) exhibit Higuchi-Diffusion model of release with t ½ 268.65 minutes. On the other hand, the release of metronidazole tablets manufactured with HPMC 15000 in drug: polymer ratio 2:1(formula 1tA) was observed to follow Hixson-Crowell model with t ½ of 208.64 minutes. Concerning metronidazole tablets containing HPMC 15000 in drug: polymer ratio 2:3 (formula 1tC), their release exhibit zero order kinetic with t ½ of 380.75 minutes. Finally, the order of release of metronidazole from its tablet with HPMC 15000 in drug: polymer ratio 1:2 (formula 1tD) was found to obey first order kinetic with t ½ of 312.78 minutes.

2-Formulae obtained using HPMC 4000

The contents of the metronidazole tablets containing different ratios of HPMC 4000 were given by Table (5a).

Table (56) and Figure (14) represent the in-vitro release of metronidazole from tablet formulae 2tA, 2tB, 2tC, and 2tD that contain HPMC 4000 in drug: polymer ratios 2:1, 1:1, 2:3, and 1:2 respectively. It is clear that by changing the viscosity grade of the same polymer type (exchange HPMC 15000 cp with HPMC 4000 cp) the release rate for all the formulae increased by decreasing the molecular weight of the polymer HPMC. These results were in accordance with the conclusion of Gerogiannis et al., (1993), who reported that higher viscosity grades of the same polymer display significant slower rates of polymer hydration. The maximum and minimum in-vitro release after 6 hours of dissolution from metronidazole formulae containing HPMC 4000 was found to be equal to 100% and 91.7% concerning formula 2tB(drug: polymer ratio 1:1) and formula 2tD (drug: polymer ratio 1:2), respectively .

The investigated tablet formulae containing metronidazole with HPMC 4000 in different drug: polymer ratios can be arranged, in ascending way, concerning dissolution rate of metronidazole, as follows: 2tD (drug: polymer ratio 1:2), 2tC(drug: polymer ratio 2:3), 2tB(drug: polymer ratio 1:1), and finally 2tA(drug: polymer ratio 2:1).

The kinetic analysis of the release data of metronidazole from its tablets containing different ratios of HPMC 4000 showed in Table (57).

167

At the pH of the dissolution medium 1.2, the diffusion controlled equation gave, for most of the formulae (2tA, 2t B, and 2tD), higher value for the correlation coefficient than did the other applied parameters of kinetic analysis. They show t ½ values of 479.48, 120.05, and 114.9 minutes, respectively. In this case the existence of the release linearly correlated to the square root of time was in agreement with the use of the HPMC 4000, which is a gel forming hydrocolloid. The drug was slowly released by diffusion through the gelatinous barrier (Ingani et al., 1987 and Gerogiannis et al., 1993).This was with the exception of formula 2tc (drug: polymer ratio 2:3) which showed a first order release with t ½ value of 101.66 minutes.

3-Formulae obtained using Carbopol 934

The contents of metronidazole tablets containing Carbopol 934 with different ratios were given in Table (5a).The in-vitro release of metronidazole from its tablets containing different ratios of Carbopol 934 was showed in Table (58) and illustrated in Figure (15).

The maximum and minimum percent released was 100% and 73.2% for metronidazole tablets containing Carbopol 934 with drug: polymer ratio 4:1 (formula 3tF) and metronidazole tablet containing Carbopol 934 in drug: polymer ratio 1:2 (formula 3tD) after 2.5, and 6 hours, respectively.

The investigated tablet formulae containing metronidazole and Carbopol 934 in different drug: polymer ratios can be arranged, in ascending order, regarding the dissolution rate of metronidazole, as follows: formula 3tF (drug: polymer ratio 4:1), formula 3tE (drug: polymer 3:1), formula

168

3tA(drug: polymer ratio 2:1), 3tB(drug: polymer ratio 1:1), formula 3tC(drug: polymer ratio2:3), and finally formula 3tD (drug: polymer ratio 1:2).

Table (59) represents the kinetic analysis of the release data of metronidazole from its tablet containing different ratios of Carbopol 934.

It is clear that, the drug release from formulae 3tC (drug: polymer ratio 2:3) and 3tE (drug: polymer ratio 3:1) followed the Higuchi model of diffusion with t ½ values of 210.66 and 60.96 minutes, respectively. In contrast, formula 3tA (drug: polymer ratio 2:1) was observed to follow Hixson-Crowell model with t ½ value of 155.78 minutes. Tablets of metronidazole contain Carbopol 934 in drug: polymer ratio 1:1 (formula 3tB) was found to obey first order kinetic with t ½ value of 216.27 minutes. While metronidazole tablet containing Carbopol 934 in drug: polymer ratio of 1:2 (formula 3tD) showed zero order release with t ½ value of 423.11 minutes. The order of release of metronidazole from its tablets containing Carbopol 934 with drug: polymer ratio 4:1 (formula 3tF) was observed to follow Baker and Lansdale equation with t ½ value of 16.39 minutes.

4-Formulae containing Na alginate

The contents of metronidazole tablets containing Na alginate with different ratios were given in Table (5a).

Table (60) and Figure (16) showed the in-vitro release of metronidazole from its tablets prepared with different ratios of Na alginate in dissolution medium of 0.1N HCl pH 1.2. The maximum and minimum in-vitro release of metronidazole was found to be 100% and 78% from formula

4tD (drug: polymer ratio 1:2) and formula 4tC (drug: polymer ratio 2:3) after about 2, and 6 hours respectively.

The investigated tablet formulae containing metronidazole and Na alginate in different drug: polymer ratios can be arranged, regarding the increase in the release of metronidazole, as follows: formula 4tC (drug: polymer ratio 2:3), formula 4tB (drug: polymer 1:1), formula 4tA (drug: polymer ratio 2:1), and finally 4tD (drug: polymer ratio 1:2). The increase in the release of the drug from tablets prepared with Na alginate than those prepared with HPMC polymers may be attributed to the fact that alginate matrices generally deliver low molecular weight drugs quickly as reported by several papers (Tanaka et al., 1984, Kim and Lee 1992).

The release of the drug from formulae containing Na alginate in different ratios was shown in Table (61) with the kinetic analysis of the release data.

It is clear from the table, that the predominance in the drug release from formulae 4tA (drug: polymer ratio 2:1), 4tB (drug: polymer ratio 1:1), and 4tD (drug: polymer ratio 1:2) follow the zero order kinetic with t ½ values of 627.49, 248.419 and 65.0759 minutes, respectively. Formula 4tC (drug: polymer ratio 2:3) was found to obey Higuchi-Diffusion model of release with t ½ value of 211.898 minutes.

5- Formulae containing Carboxymethyl cellulose (CMC)

The contents of metronidazole tablets containing CMC with different drug: polymer ratios were given in Table (5b).

170

The in-vitro release of metronidazole from its tablet containing different ratios of CMC was showed in Table (62) and illustrated in Figure (17).The maximum and minimum percent released was 100% and 77.6% after 5.5, and 6 hours from metronidazole tablets containing CMC with drug: polymer ratio 2:1 (formula 5tA) and metronidazole tablet containing CMC in drug: polymer ratio 1:2 (formula 5tD), respectively.

The investigated tablet formulae containing metronidazole and CMC in different drug: polymer ratios can be arranged, in ascending order, regarding the dissolution rate of metronidazole, as follows: formula 5tD (drug: polymer ratio 1:2), formula 5tB (drug: polymer 1:1), formula 5tC(drug: polymer ratio 2:3), and finally formula 5tA (drug: polymer ratio 2:1).

Table (63) represents the kinetic analysis of the release data of metronidazole from its tablet containing different ratios of CMC.

It is clear that, the diffusion controlled equation gave, for most of formulae (5tA, 5tB, and 5tC), high values for the correlation coefficient than other applied kinetic parameters with t ½ values of 230.17, 166.23, and 88.98 minutes, respectively. This was in exception of formula 5tD which showed zero order release with t ½ value of 170.257 minutes.

6-Formulae containing Ethyl cellulose
The contents of metronidazole tablet containing ethyl cellulose with different ratios were given in Table (5b).

171

Plots of percent metronidazole released from its tablets containing different ratios of ethyl cellulose, with time are shown in Table (64) and illustrated in Figure (18). It is clear that those tablets containing ethyl cellulose in drug: polymer ratios 1:1 (formula 6tB), 2:3 (formula 6tC) and 1:2 (formula 6tD) reach the maximum release of 100% after two hours of dissolution. Whereas, those tablets containing ethyl cellulose in drug: polymer ratio 2:1 (formula 6tA) showed faster release of their drug content and reach maximum release of 100% after only one hour.

Table (65) represents the kinetic analysis of the release data of metronidazole from its tablet containing different ratios of ethyl cellulose.

It is clear from the table, that zero order kinetic controlled the release of metronidazole from its tablets containing ethyl cellulose in drug: polymer ratios 1:1(formula 6tB), drug: polymer ratio 2:3 (formula 6tC) and drug: polymer ratio 1:2 (formula 6tD) with t ½ values of 592.88, 576.9 and 429.79 minutes, respectively. Concerning metronidazole tablets containing ethyl cellulose in drug: polymer ratio 2:1 (formula 6tA), they followed the Higuchi model of diffusion with t ½ value of 5949.8 minutes.

7-Formulae containing Methyl cellulose

The contents of metronidazole tablet containing methyl cellulose with different ratios were showed in Table (5b).

Plot of percent metronidazole released from its tablet contain different ratios of methyl cellulose with time are shown in Table (66) and illustrated in Figure (19). The maximum and minimum in-vitro release of

172

metronidazole after 6 hours of dissolution was found to be 93.1% and 83.7% from formula 7tA (drug: polymer ratio 2:1) and formula 7tD (drug: polymer ratio 1:2), respectively.

The investigated tablet formulae containing metronidazole and methyl cellulose in different drug: polymer ratios can be arranged, in ascending manner, regarding the dissolution rate of metronidazole, as follows: formula 7tD (drug: polymer ratio 1:2), formula 7tC (drug: polymer 2:3), formula 7tB (drug: polymer ratio 1:1), and finally 7tA (drug: polymer ratio 2:1).

Table (67) represents the kinetic analysis of the release data of metronidazole from its tablet containing different ratios of methyl cellulose.

It is obvious that, formula 7tB (drug: polymer ratio 1:1) and formula 7tC (drug: polymer ratio 2:3) followed first order kinetic with t ½ values of 117.07, and 158.319 minutes, respectively. Regarding formula 7tA (drug: polymer ratio 2:1) was found to obey Hixson-Crowell model with t ½ value of 131.93 minutes. On the other hand formula 7tD (drug: polymer ratio 1:2) was observed to follow Baker and Lansdale equation with t ½ value of 93.139 minutes.

8-Formulae obtained using Pectin

The contents of metronidazole tablet containing pectin with different ratios were given in Table (5b).

Table (68) and Figure (20) demonstrate the difference between metronidazole release profiles from its tablets prepared with different ratios

173

of pectin. The maximum in-vitro release of metronidazole was found to be 100% after 1 hour from both formulae 8tA and 8tB (drug: polymer ratio 2:1 and 1:1) while formula 8tG (drug: polymer ratio 1:3) gave the minimum release of the drug (76.3%) after 6 hours.

The investigated metronidazole tablet formulae containing pectin in different drug: polymer ratios can be arranged, in ascending manner, regarding the dissolution rate of metronidazole, as follows: both formulae 8tA (drug: polymer ratio 2:1) & formula 8tB (drug: polymer 1:1), then formula 8tC (drug: polymer ratio 2:3), then formula8t (drug: polymer ratio 1:2) and finally 8tG (drug: polymer ratio 1:3).

Table (69) demonstrates the kinetic analysis of the release data of metronidazole from its tablet containing different ratios of pectin in simulated gastric medium.

It is apparent that from the table, the metronidazole tablet containing pectin in drug: polymer ratios 2:1 and 1:1 exhibit zero order kinetic with t ½ values of 66.964, and 65.5 minutes, respectively. While, those metronidazole tablets containing pectin in drug: polymer ratios of 2:3 and 1:3 follow Higuchi-Diffusion model with t ½ values of 73.206, and 122.28 minutes respectively. At last, the order of release of metronidazole tablets containing pectin with drug: polymer ratio1:2 was observed to follow Hixson-Crowell model with t ½ value of 122.28 minutes.

In order to compare the in-vitro release of metronidazole tablets using different ratios of different polymers, the data obtained for the same drug:

polymer ratio concerning the eight polymers employed was estimated, to compare the retardation effect of each polymer on metronidazole.

In-vitro release of metronidazole from the formulated tablets using different polymers with the same drug: polymer ratio 2:1 was showed in Table (70) and Figure (21). The minimum in-vitro release was 73% for metronidazole tablets containing HPMC 15000 after 6 hours. The retardation of metronidazole release from tablets was arranged, in ascending order, as follow: HPMC 15000 (formula 1tA) >Carbopol 934 (formula 3tA) > Methyl cellulose (formula 7tA) > CMC (formula 5tA) > HPMC 4000 (formula 2tA) & Na alginate (formula 4tA) > ethyl cellulose (formula 6tA) and pectin (formula 8tA).

Table (71) and Figure (22) demonstrates the difference between metronidazole release profiles from metronidazole tablets prepared with different polymer in drug: polymer ratio 1:1. The minimum in-vitro release was 66.5% for formula 1tB (containing HPMC 15000). The retardation of metronidazole tablets was arranged, in ascending manner, as follows: HPMC 15000 (formula 1tB) > Carbopol 934 (formula 3tB) > methyl cellulose (formula 7tB) > CMC (formula 5tB) > HPMC 4000 (formula 2tB) & Na alginate (formula 4tB) > ethyl cellulose (formula 6tB) > pectin (formula 8tB).

The in-vitro release of metronidazole from its tablets prepared with different polymers with the drug: polymer ratio 2:3 was observed in Table (72) and Figure (23).The minimum in-vitro release was 64.2% belonged to metronidazole tablets containing HPMC 15000. The retardation of

175

metronidazole tablets was arranged, in ascending mode, as follows: HPMC 15000 (formula 1tC) > Carbopol 934 (formula 3tC) > Na alginate (formula 4tC) > methyl cellulose (formula 7tC) > HPMC 4000 (formula 2tC) > CMC (formula 5tC) > ethyl cellulose (formula 6tC) >pectin (formula 8tC).

The in-vitro release of metronidazole from its tablets prepared with different polymers with the drug: polymer ratio 1:2 was observed in Table (73) and Figure (24).The minimum in-vitro release was 59.2% concerning metronidazole tablets containing HPMC 15000. The retardation of metronidazole tablets was arranged, in ascending manner, as follows: HPMC 15000 (formula 1tD) > Carbopol 934 (formula 3tD) > CMC (formula 5tD) > methyl cellulose (formula 7tD) > pectin (formula 8tD) > HPMC 4000 (formula 2tD) > Na alginate (formula 4tD) & ethyl cellulose (formula 6tD).

Regarding the release of metronidazole from its tablets prepared with same ingredient showed in Table (5a) but with no polymers by direct compression technique (plain tablet) in the same dissolution medium, was illustrated in all previous in-vitro release Tables as contrast with other tablet formulae. The plain tablets evoked a very high release at pH 1.2 as they release about 81% of their drug content after 30 minutes at the same time the entire drug content was released after 60 minutes. These findings comply with the USP (2000) requirements which stated that not less than 85% of the labeled amount of metronidazole to be dissolved in one hour.

While the data which showed the kinetic treatment of the in-vitro release of metronidazole from its directly compressed plain tablets were illustrated in all previous kinetic tables of other tablet formulae. It can be

176

observed that the order of release of metronidazole from its plain tablets followed Higuchi model of diffusion with t ½ value of 104.45 minutes.

Finally, from the previous in-vitro release profile of metronidazole from its slow-release tablets prepared by direct compression technique, it can be concluded that formulae 1tA (metronidazole tablet containing HPMC 15000 in drug: polymer ratio 2:1), 2tC (metronidazole tablet containing HPMC 4000 in drug: polymer ratio 2:3), 3tA (metronidazole tablet containing Carbopol 934 in drug: polymer ratio 2:1), 5tB (metronidazole tablet containing CMC in drug: polymer ratio 1:1), 7tA (metronidazole tablet containing methyl cellulose in drug: polymer ratio 2:1), and 8tD (metronidazole tablet containing pectin in drug: polymer ratio 1:2), be able to deliver metronidazole at constant rate up to 90% of the total loading dose during 6 hours dissolution. So, those formulae were prepared as two-layer floating tablets. The first layer provided floating which contained the mixture of sodium bicarbonate and calcium carbonate (ratio 1:2) and hydroxylpropyl methyl cellulose 4000 .The second layer (release layer) provided the previous controlled release metronidazole tablet formula.

Floating dosage forms with an in situ gas generating mechanism are expected to have greater buoyancy and improved drug release characteristics. However, the optimization of the drug release may alter the buoyancy and therefore, it is necessary to separate the control of buoyancy from that of drug release kinetics during formulation optimization (Rouge et al., 1996).

In-vitro buoyancy lag time and floating capacity optimization of prepared metronidazole tablets were shown in Tables (74 and 75) and illustrated in Figures (25 and 26). It has been reported that floating delivery systems can prolong the gastric retention time and thus increase the overall drug bioavailability for certain drugs (Ingani et al., 1987; Timmermans and Moes 1994; Erni and Held 1987; Moes 1993). In this work, for greater localized effect of metronidazole tablets, the floating strategy was taken into consideration in the design of delivery system. The buoyancy of prepared tablets was accomplished by incorporating gas-generating salt sodium bicarbonate and calcium carbonate into a swellable hydrophilic layer (HPMC 4000). The overall makeup of this particular matrix is of swellable hydrophilic polymers. As the dissolution medium was imbedded into the matrix, the interaction of acidic fluid (0.1 N HCl) with sodium bicarbonate/calcium carbonate resulted in the formation and entrapment of CO_2 gas within the swollen gel thus causing floatation as the matrix volume expanded and its density decreased see Figure (27).

It is observed that the buoyancy lag time for this system is in the range of 3-60 minutes and no floatation was achieved below the minimum gas-generating quantity of 7.5 mg. Also the system was float over the entire dissolution period in each case. The result implied that the thickness of gas-generating layer can vary over a wide range and as a result the desired release duration can easily achieved. Since larger tablets might have the potential to stay in stomach for a longer time period (Moes, 1993), in this work, maximum amount of gas-generating mixture (60 mg) which show the lowest lag floating time (3 minutes) was incorporated into the gas-generating layer. So it was not worthy behavior of all the prepared formulae as there

178

was no significant difference in the floating behavior among them and they all showed floating time of about 6 hour

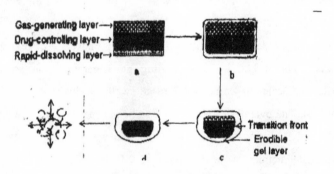

Figure (27): Schematic representation of the macroscopic changes associated with bilayer tablet delivery system during dissolution study. a, initial configuration of the system; b, after introduction into the dissolution medium the matrix start swelling; c, system dynamics of swelling and erosion; d, and e, system erosion leading to complete dissolution (Libo et al., 1999).

179

CONCLUSION

From the previous results and discussion the following could be concluded:

1-All the prepared metronidazole tablets manufactured by directly compression technique complied with the pharmacopoeial requirements for uniformity of weight, thickness, drug content, and disintegration time, while have reasonable hardness and friability values.

2-Conventional slow-release tablets of metronidazole were designed to provide almost linear and complete drug release within 6 hours. Formulae 1tA (metronidazole tablet containing HPMC 15000 in drug: polymer ratio 2:1), 2tC (metronidazole tablet containing HPMC 4000 in drug: polymer ratio 2:3), 3tA (metronidazole tablet containing Carbopol 934 in drug: polymer ratio 2:1), 5tB (metronidazole tablet containing CMC in drug: polymer ratio 1:1), 7tA (metronidazole tablet containing methyl cellulose in drug: polymer ratio 2:1), and 8tD (metronidazole tablet containing pectin in drug: polymer ratio 1:2), were be able to deliver the drug at constant rates up to 90% of the total loading dose.

3-Stable and persistent buoyancy of metronidazole bilayer tablets was achieved by trapping the gas in the gel formed by the hydration of hydroxyl propyl methyl cellulose 4000.

4-It is observed that the buoyancy lag time for this bilayer tablet system is in range 3-60 minutes according to the weight of gas-generating mixture.

5-The prepared bilayer tablet be able to float over the entire dissolution period (6 hours) in all investigated weight of gas-generating layer.

6- The in-vitro release of metronidazole from the investigated tablets followed different kinetic orders and no one kinetic order can express the drug release.

This chapter showed an intragastric floating of the two-layer tablet of metronidazole to remain in the stomach for a longer time. This developed delivery system increased the efficacy of the therapy for Helicobacter pylori associated ulcers and improved patient compliance.

CHAPTER II

NON-EFFEREVESCENT METRONIDAZOLE FLOATING PREPARATIONS

Introduction

A floating dosage unit is useful for drugs acting locally in the proximal gastrointestinal tract. These systems are also useful for drugs which are poorly soluble or unstable in intestinal fluids. The floating properties of these systems help in retaining these systems in the stomach for a long time. Various attempts have been made to develop a floating system. This system will float on gastric contents for a desired time period. During this time period drug will be released from this system. After the release of the drug, the remnants of the system will be emptied from the stomach.

The first report of a floating dosage form designed for sustained drug delivery was in 1975, when Sheth and Tossounian, 1979 published a patent for a hydrodynamically balanced system (HBS). The unit consists of capsule formulation containing the drug, hydrocolloids, and various other excipeints. After immersion in aqueous media, the capsule dissolves, and the hydrocolloid forms a hydrated boundary layer that gives the formulation its floating properties. The drug subsequently is released through this layer by diffusion. Progressive erosion of the outer gelled boundary layer allows hydration and gelation of exposed inner layers, maintaining the diffusion barrier and floating ability.

Since then several approaches have been used to develop an ideal floating delivery system, include non effervescent and effervescent systems. The most commonly used excipeints in noneffervescent floating drug delivery system are gel-forming or highly swellable cellulose type hydrocolloids, polycarbonate, and matrix forming polymers such as polycarbonate, polyacrylate, polymethacrylate and polystyrene.

All floating dosage forms have the common property of possessing a density lower than that of gastric fluids. In some systems, hydration must occur before this criterion is fulfilled and lag times before buoyancy are apparent. Both the desired time period for buoyancy and the rate of drug release can be modulated by the appropriate selection of a polymer matrix.

This chapter investigate development of non effervescent floating preparations of locally acting metronidazole including preparation of single-unit systems (floating capsules), and multiple-unit systems (floating hollow microspheres or microballoons).The in vitro release of metronidazole from the different preparations prepared with different ratios of various polymers as well as the various approaches used in and their mechanism of buoyancy are discussed in the following chapter.

For comparison purpose, immediate release reference capsules and microspheres containing the same dose of metronidazole were also formulated.

The prepared capsules were evaluated for their uniformity of drug content. As well as the microspheres prepared were physically evaluated for their particle size and morphology. The kinetic parameters for the in-vitro release of metronidazole were determined and analyzed in order to explain the mechanism of drug release. Specific computer program was used for this purpose.

184

Experimental

Material:

- Metronidazole powder, poly vinyl alcohol, and Eudragit S100, kindly supplied by Egyptian International Pharmaceutical Industries Company (E.I.P.I.Co), Egypt.
- Microcrystalline cellulose (Avicel pH 101), Pectin (USP), Aerosil 200, starch 1500, kindly supplied by El-Nile Pharmaceutical-Chemical Company, Cairo, Egypt.
- Methyl cellulose, Hydroxypropyl methylcellulose (HPMC) 4000 and 15000 cps grades, Na alginate, Carbopol 934, and carboxy methylcellulose (CMC), kindly supplied by El-Kahira Pharmaceutical-Chemical Company, Cairo, Egypt.
- Absolute ethanol, Isopropyl alcohol, and dichloromethane, of pure analytical grade, Adwic, Egypt.
- Hydrochloric acid, specific gravity 1.16 GPR), El-Nasr Chemicals Company, Cairo, Egypt.
- Ethyl cellulose, Fluka, (Switzerland).
- Hard gelatin capsules size number (00), kindly supplied by Egyptian International Pharmaceutical Industries Company (E.I.P.I.Co), Egypt.

Equipment:

- Electric balance: Mettler, J100, (Switzerland).
- Spectrophotometer, Jenway LTD: Model: 610 suvlvis, (England).
- Modified USP dissolution tester (Scientific). DA.6D, Bombay-400-069, (India).
- Mechanical stirrer (M.S.E. Homogeniser), (England).

Methodology:

1-Construction of the standard calibration curve of metronidazole:
The same as in chapter I.

2-Development of Non effervescent floating preparations of metronidazole
2.1-Preparation of Sustained Release Floating Capsule of metronidazole (SRFC):
Metronidazole: polymer (HPMC 15000, HPMC 4000, Na alginate, Carbopol 934, Pectin, Ethyl cellulose, Methyl cellulose and CMC) ratios of 2:1, 1:1, 2:3 and 1:2 were used primarily to formulate the sustained release of metronidazole over 6 hours. Aerosil was used in concentration 0.4% w/w as a lubricant. Avicel was used as adjuvant in quantities so as to be sufficient to fill a hard gelatin capsule size 00.

The calculated amounts of powdered ingredients for each formula mentioned in Tables (78-85) were simply mixed in a large dish until a homogenous mixture was obtained which is then filled volumetrically as non compressed powder by means of manual filling method into the hard gelatin capsule size 00.

The bulk density of metronidazole, polymers (HPMC 15000, HPMC 4000, Pectin, CMC, Na alginate, Methyl cellulose, Ethyl cellulose and Carbopol 934), Avicel pH 101 and Aerosil 200 was determined by using plastic syringes (Abd.Hameed,1996). Suitable weight of each ingredient was filled separately in the syringe. The corresponding volume was determined. The bulk density of the ingredient was then calculated by dividing the ingredient weight by its corresponding volume. The results were illustrated in Table (76).

2.2-Preparation of Sustained Release Floating Microspheres (SRFM) of Metronidazole:

Microspheres with an internal hollow structure were prepared by a modified emulsion solvent diffusion and evaporation method.

Typically, 0.25, 0.5, and 1 g of Eudragit S100 with 0.5 g of metronidazole were dissolved in 8 ml ethanol, followed by the addition of 2 ml isopropanol and 5 ml dichloromethane. This solution was slowly introduced by a syringe (Dalia, 2002) into 500 ml aqueous solution of 0.4% polyvinyl alcohol with stirring at 250 rpm using a mechanical stirrer equipped with a 3-blade propeller. The solution was stirred for 10 minutes and the microspheres were collected by filtration. The collected microspheres were dried for 12 hours at 50°C.

Plain microspheres devoid of drug to be used as blank sample were also prepared by the same previous method.

3-Dissolution testing for the sustained release floating preparations of metronidazole:

The release of metronidazole from the prepared both floating microspheres and floating capsules was done using the USP rotating basket method (type I). The dissolution media consisted of 900 ml simulated gastric fluid (pH 1.2) maintained at $37\pm0.5°C$ and the rotation at 50 rotation per minute.

One capsule of each formulated metronidazole sustained release floating system (each contains 125 mg metronidazole) was placed in each of the three dissolution vessels. Microspheres from each formulae equivalent to 125 mg of metronidazole were also subjected to the dissolution testing. Each dissolution test was composed of three tests and blank samples. The blank in case of metronidazole microspheres was mad using microballoons containing the same ingredients without metronidazole.

At specified time intervals; 5ml sample was withdrawn from each of the six dissolution media and filtered off. Clear sample was withdrawn from each filtrate and measured spectrophotometrically at 278 nm against the corresponding blank. The dissolution volume was kept constant all over the dissolution time, by compensation of the withdrawn volume.

The percentage metronidazole release was calculated and the mean of three experiments was determined. Mean results were tabulated and graphically illustrated in Tables (94, 96, 98, 100, 102, 104, 106, and 108) and figures (29-36). The dissolution data was also subjected to a series of computerized statistical, mathematical and kinetic calculations. Results are shown in Tables (95, 97, 99, 101, 103, 105, 107, and 109).

4- Dissolution testing for plain metronidazole preparations:

The dissolution profile of plain metronidazole capsules (capsule containing 125mg metronidazole without addition of any polymers) was determined by the USP rotating basket method (type I).Also the dissolution profile of plain drug (125 mg metronidazole without any additions) was performed for comparison purpose regarding metronidazole microspheres.

The dissolution test procedures were done as mentioned before. The percentage metronidazole release was calculated and the mean of three experiments was determined.

5-Floating time and floating properties:

a-For capsules dosage forms:

The same USP dissolution apparatus was used in this test after removing the basket. Each of the six glass vessels of the apparatus was filled with 900 ml of simulated gastric fluid of pH1.2 and all maintained at 37±0.5°C.Each formula was tested separately by placing in the solution. The time between the introduction of the dosage form into the dissolution medium and its buoyancy to the top of dissolution medium was the buoyancy lag time and the duration of system floatation was observed visually and tabulated in Tables (114-121) and was shown as histogram in Figure (41).

b-For metronidazole floating microsphere preparations:

The same USP dissolution apparatus was used in this test. Each of the six glass vessels of the apparatus was filled with 900 ml of simulated gastric fluid of pH1.2 and all maintained at 37±0.5°C. Each formula was tested separately by placing in the solution. Microspheres were spread over the surface of the medium. A paddle was adjusted at 50 rpm. Microspheres floating on the surface were collected at a predetermined time (after 6 hours). The collected sample was weighed after drying. Results are shown in Table (124).

6-Charactrizations of prepared metronidazole dosage forms:
6.1- Capsules dosage form:

6.1.1-Testing the uniformity of drug content:

Ten different capsules from each formula were mixed. Samples of 500 mg were tested for drug content as adopted in chapter I. The mean drug content percent, standard deviation and coefficient of variation percent were calculated. Results are shown in Tables (86-92) and shown as histogram in Figure (28).

6.2- Metronidazole floating microsphere preparations:

6.2.1-Yield of microspheres formation:

The each formula of prepared microspheres were collected, dried and weighed. The measured weight was divided by the total amount components used for the preparation of the microspheres (drug + polymer) as shown in Table (124).

6.2.2-Loading efficiency:

An amount of prepared microspheres were weighed and dissolved in 100 ml 0.1N HCl to measure the amount of drug loaded spectrophotometrically at 278 nm. This value will equal to the actual drug content.

The loading efficiency was calculated by dividing actual drug content over theoretical drug content as shown in Table (124).

6.2.3-Uniformity of drug content:

From the dried microspheres three different samples from each formula each weighing 100 mg were tested for drug content as follows:

The microspheres of each sample were extracted with successive portion of 0.1 N HCl and then filtered in volumetric flask 100 ml. The filtration was continued until 100 ml of each sample was collected. Plain microspheres devoid of drug were extracted as the previous method. Then the three samples were measured for drug content spectrophotometrically at 278 nm using plain microspheres extract as blank.

No significant difference was found among the three tested samples indicating uniformity of drug content.

6.2.4-Particle size analysis:

The particle size distribution of the microspheres was measured by the sieve analysis. The range of sieves employed ranged from (1000-90) µm. The sieve analysis of each formula of metronidazole microspheres were represented in Table (125).

6.2.5-Morphology:

The morphology and surface characteristics of the microspheres were examined by a scanning electric microscope. The photomicrographs of microspheres were shown in Figures (43-45).

Table (76): The estimated bulk density of metronidazole of different formulations.

Material	weight of powder (g)	Corresponding volume of powder (cm^3)	Bulk density (g/cm^3)
Metronidazole	2.5	2.8	0.89
HPMC 15000	2.5	4.6	0.54
HPMC 4000	2.5	3.4	0.73
Na alginate	2.5	2.6	0.96
Carbopol 934	2.5	8.5	0.29
CMC	2.5	4.4	0.56
Ethyl cellulose	2.5	4.8	0.52
Methyl cellulose	2.5	4.7	0.53
Pectin	2.5	3.4	0.73
Avicel	2.5	5.5	0.45
Aerosil	0.852	7.8	0.11

Table (77): The prepared formulae of metronidazole capsules using different polymers.

Formulae	Polymer	Drug: polymer ratio
1cA	HPMC 15000	2:1
1cB	HPMC 15000	1:1
1cC	HPMC 15000	2:3
1cD	HPMC 15000	1:2
2cA	HPMC 4000	2:1
2cB	HPMC 4000	1:1
2cC	HPMC 4000	2:3
2cD	HPMC 4000	1:2
3cA	Carbopol 934	2:1
3cB	Carbopol 934	1:1
3cC	Carbopol 934	2:3
3cD	Carbopol 934	1:2
4cA	Na alginate	2:1
4cB	Na alginate	1:1
4cC	Na alginate	2:3
4cD	Na alginate	1:2
5cA	CMC	2:1
5cB	CMC	1:1
5cC	CMC	2:3
5cD	CMC	1:2
6cA	Ethyl cellulose	2:1
6cB	Ethyl cellulose	1:1
6cC	Ethyl cellulose	2:3
6cD	Ethyl cellulose	1:2
7cA	Methyl cellulose	2:1
7cB	Methyl cellulose	1:1
7cC	Methyl cellulose	2:3
7cD	Methyl cellulose	1:2
8cA	Pectin	2:1
8cB	Pectin	1:1
8cC	Pectin	2:3
8cD	Pectin	1:2

Table (78): Formulation of metronidazole floating capsules using HPMC 15000 with different drug: polymer ratios.

Ingredients	Formulae weight in mg				Formulae volume in cm^3			
	1cA	1cB	1cC	1cD	1cA	1cB	1cC	1cD
Metronidazole	125	125	125	125	0.14	0.14	0.14	0.14
HPMC15000	62.5	125	187.5	250	0.11	0.23	0.345	0.46
Aerosil	2	2	2	2	0.018	0.018	0.018	0.018
Avicel	310.5	248	185.5	123	0.68	0.55	0.41	0.27
Total weight or volume	500	500	500	500	0.948	0.94	0.913	0.888

1; HPMC 15000   c; capsule dosage form

A; drug: polymer ratio 2:1   B; drug: polymer ratio 1:1

C; drug: polymer ratio 2:3   D; drug: polymer ratio 1:2

Table (79): Formulation of metronidazole floating capsules using HPMC 4000 with different drug: polymer ratios.

Ingredients	Formulae weight in mg				Formulae volume in cm^3			
	2cA	2cB	2cC	2cD	2cA	2cB	2cC	2cD
Metronidazole	125	125	125	125	0.14	0.14	0.14	0.14
HPMC 4000	62.5	125	187.5	250	0.105	0.17	0.255	0.34
Aerosil	2	2	2	2	0.018	0.018	0.018	0.018
Avicel	310.5	248	185.5	123	0.68	0.55	0.41	0.27
Total weight or volume	500	500	500	500	0.92	0.878	0.823	0.768

2; HPMC 4000   c; capsule dosage form

A; drug: polymer ratio 2:1   B; drug: polymer ratio 1:1

C; drug: polymer ratio 2:3   D; drug: polymer ratio 1:2

Table (80): Formulation of metronidazole floating capsules using Carbopol 934 with different drug: polymer ratios.

Ingredients	Formulae weight in mg				Formulae volume in cm^3			
	3cA	3cB	3cC	3cD	3cA	3cB	3cC	3cD
Metronidazole	125	125	125	125	0.14	0.14	0.14	0.14
Carbopol 934	62.5	125	187.5	250	0.2	0.43	0.64	0.85
Aerosil	2	2	2	2	0.018	0.018	0.018	0.018
Avicel	310.5	248	185.5	123	0.68	0.55	0.41	0.27
Total weight or volume	500	500	500	500	1.038	1.138	1.208	1.278

3; Carbopol 934   c; capsule dosage form

A; drug: polymer ratio 2:1   B; drug: polymer ratio 1:1

C; drug: polymer ratio 2:3   D; drug: polymer ratio 1:2

Table (81): Formulation of metronidazole floating capsules using sodium alginate with different drug: polymer ratios.

Ingredients	Formulae weight in mg				Formulae volume in cm^3			
	4cA	4cB	4cC	4cD	4cA	4cB	4cC	4cD
Metronidazole	125	125	125	125	0.14	0.14	0.14	0.14
Na alginate	62.5	125	187.5	250	0.065	0.13	0.195	0.26
Aerosil	2	2	2	2	0.018	0.018	0.018	0.018
Avicel	310.5	248	185.5	123	0.68	0.55	0.41	0.27
Total weight or volume	500	500	500	500	0.903	0.838	0.76	0.688

4; Na alginate   c; capsule dosage form

A; drug: polymer ratio 2:1   B; drug: polymer ratio 1:1

C; drug: polymer ratio 2:3   D; drug: polymer ratio 1:2

Table (82): Formulation of metronidazole floating capsules using CMC with different drug: polymer ratios.

Ingredients	Formulae weight in mg				Formulae volume in cm^3			
	5cA	5cB	5cC	5cD	5cA	5cB	5cC	5cD
Metronidazole	125	125	125	125	0.14	0.14	0.14	0.14
CMC	62.5	125	187.5	250	0.11	0.22	0.33	0.44
Aerosil	2	2	2	2	0.018	0.018	0.018	0.018
Avicel	310.5	248	185.5	123	0.68	0.55	0.41	0.27
Total weight or volume	500	500	500	500	0.95	0.93	0.898	0.868

5; CMC   c; capsule dosage form

A; drug: polymer ratio 2:1   B; drug: polymer ratio 1:1

C; drug: polymer ratio 2:3   D; drug: polymer ratio 1:2

Table (83): Formulation of metronidazole floating capsules using Ethylcellulose with different drug: polymer ratios.

Ingredients	Formulae weight in mg				Formulae volume in cm^3			
	6cA	6cB	6cC	6cD	6cA	6cB	6cC	6cD
Metronidazole	125	125	125	125	0.14	0.14	0.14	0.14
Ethylcellulose	62.5	125	187.5	250	0.12	0.24	0.36	0.48
Aerosil	2	2	2	2	0.018	0.018	0.018	0.018
Avicel	310.5	248	185.5	123	0.68	0.55	0.41	0.27
Total weight or volume	500	500	500	500	0.96	0.95	0.93	0.91

6; ethyl cellulose   c; capsule dosage form

A; drug: polymer ratio 2:1   B; drug: polymer ratio 1:1

C; drug: polymer ratio 2:3   D; drug: polymer ratio 1:2

197

Table (84): Formulation of metronidazole floating capsules using Pectin with different drug: polymer ratios.

Ingredients	Formulae weight in mg				Formulae volume in cm^3			
	7cA	7cB	7cC	7cD	7cA	7cB	7cC	7cD
Metronidazole	125	125	125	125	0.14	0.14	0.14	0.14
Methylcellulose	62.5	125	187.5	250	0.12	0.24	0.35	0.47
Aerosil	2	2	2	2	0.018	0.018	0.018	0.018
Avicel	310.5	248	185.5	123	0.68	0.55	0.41	0.27
Total weight or volume	500	500	500	500	0.96	0.95	0.92	0.898

7; methyl cellulose   c; capsule dosage form

A; drug: polymer ratio 2:1   B; drug: polymer ratio 1:1

C; drug: polymer ratio 2:3   D; drug: polymer ratio 1:2

Table (85): Formulation of metronidazole floating capsules using Pectin with different drug: polymer ratios.

Ingredients	Formulae weight in mg				Formulae volume in cm^3			
	8cA	8cB	8cC	8cD	8cA	8cB	8cC	8cD
Metronidazole	125	125	125	125	0.14	0.14	0.14	0.14
Pectin	62.5	125	187.5	250	0.085	0.17	0.25	0.34
Aerosil	2	2	2	2	0.018	0.018	0.018	0.018
Avicel	310.5	248	185.5	123	0.68	0.55	0.41	0.27
Total weight or volume	500	500	500	500	0.92	0.878	0.818	0.768

8; pectin   c; capsule dosage form

A; drug: polymer ratio 2:1   B; drug: polymer ratio 1:1

C; drug: polymer ratio 2:3   D; drug: polymer ratio 1:2

Table (86): Uniformity of drug content of metronidazole capsules manufactured with different ratios of HPMC 15000.

Formula	Drug content (%)		Standard deviation	Coefficient of variation %
	mean	range		
1cA	102.4	100-106	2.8	2.7
1cB	98.2	97-99	0.8	0.81
1cC	97.2	95-99	1.6	1.6
1cD	100.4	98-101	1.1	1.1

1: polymer HPMC 15000   c: Capsule dosage form
A: drug: polymer ratio 2:1   B: drug: polymer ratio 1:1
C: drug: polymer ratio 2:3   D: drug: polymer ratio 1:2

Table (87): Uniformity of drug content of metronidazole capsules manufactured with different ratios of HPMC 4000.

Formula	Drug content (%)		Standard deviation	Coefficient of variation %
	mean	range		
2cA	99.4	98-101	1.3	1.31
2cB	99.8	98-103	2.1	2.1
2cC	97.2	95-99	1.78	1.78
2cD	94.3	92-98	2.58	2.73

2: polymer HPMC 4000   c: Capsule dosage form
A: drug: polymer ratio 2:1   B: drug: polymer ratio 1:1
C: drug: polymer ratio 2:3   D: drug: polymer ratio 1:2

Table (88): Uniformity of drug content of metronidazole capsules prepared with different ratios of Carbopol 934.

Formula	Drug content (%)		Standard deviation	Coefficient of variation %
	mean	range		
3cA	93.4	92-94.5	0.96	1.03
3cB	96.1	94.5-99	1.88	1.95
3cC	97.9	95.5-100	2.0	2.04
3cD	100.2	98-102	1.6	1.6

3: polymer Carbopol 934   c: Capsule dosage form
A: drug: polymer ratio 2:1   B: drug: polymer ratio 1:1
C: drug: polymer ratio 2:3   D: drug: polymer ratio 1:2

Table (89): Uniformity of drug content of metronidazole capsules prepared with different ratios of sodium alginate.

Formula	Drug content (%)		Standard deviation	Coefficient of variation %
	mean	range		
4cA	99.5	97-102	2.0	2.01
4cB	100.5	98-103	2.0	1.99
4cC	93.4	92-95	1.14	1.22
4cD	96.2	92-100	3.3	3.4

4: polymer Na alginate   c: Capsule dosage form
A: drug: polymer ratio 2:1   B: drug: polymer ratio 1:1
C: drug: polymer ratio 2:3   D: drug: polymer ratio 1:2

Table (90): Uniformity of drug content of metronidazole capsules prepared with different ratios of CMC.

Formula	Drug content (%)		Standard deviation	Coefficient of variation %
	mean	range		
5cA	92.6	90-95	2.3	2.48
5cB	95.6	93-98	2.4	2.51
5cC	99.8	97-102	1.9	1.9
5cD	97.2	92-101	3.96	4.07

5: polymer CMC c: Capsule dosage form
A: drug: polymer ratio 2:1 B: drug: polymer ratio 1:1
C: drug: polymer ratio 2:3 D: drug: polymer ratio 1:2

Table (91): Uniformity of drug content of metronidazole capsules prepared with different ratios of Ethyl cellulose.

Formula	Drug content (%)		Standard deviation	Coefficient of variation %
	mean	range		
6cA	97.4	93-100	3.2	3.28
6cB	93.8	92-95	1.3	1.38
6cC	96.0	93-99	2.82	2.9
6cD	99.2	97-100	1.3	1.31

6: polymer Ethyl cellulose c: Capsule dosage form
A: drug: polymer ratio 2:1 B: drug: polymer ratio 1:1
C: drug: polymer ratio 2:3 D: drug: polymer ratio 1:2

Table (92): Uniformity of drug content of metronidazole capsules prepared with different ratios of Methyl cellulose.

Formula	Drug content (%)		Standard deviation	Coefficient of variation %
	mean	range		
7cA	93.6	92-96	1.80	1.90
7cB	97.0	95-99	1.58	1.63
7cC	99.8	98-101	1.30	1.30
7cD	95.4	93-99	2.1	2.2

7: polymer Methyl cellulose   c: Capsule dosage form
A: drug: polymer ratio 2:1   B: drug: polymer ratio 1:1
C: drug: polymer ratio 2:3   D: drug: polymer ratio 1:2

Table (93): Uniformity of drug content of metronidazole capsules prepared with different ratios of Pectin.

Formula	Drug content (%)		Standard deviation	Coefficient of variation %
	mean	range		
8cA	100	98-102	1.58	1.58
8cB	97.3	95-100	2.14	2.19
8cC	94.2	93-96	1.15	1.22
8cD	92.6	91-95	1.52	1.64

8: polymer Pectin   c: Capsule dosage form
A: drug: polymer ratio 2:1   B: drug: polymer ratio 1:1
C: drug: polymer ratio 2:3   D: drug: polymer ratio 1:2

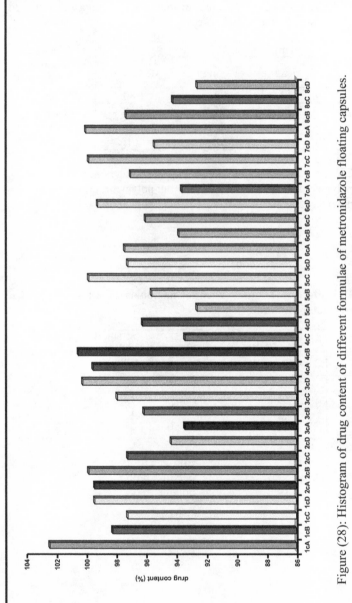

Figure (28): Histogram of drug content of different formulae of metronidazole floating capsules.

A, B, C, D; drug: polymer ratios 2:1, 1:1, 2:3, 1:2, respectively.

1,2,3,4,5,6,7,8 polymers HPMC 15000, HPMC 4000, Carbopol 934, sodium alginate, CMC, ethyl cellulose, methyl cellulose, and pectin , respectively.

Table (94): In-vitro release of metronidazole from its capsules containing HPMC 15000 in different drug: polymer ratios.

Dissolution medium	Time (hour)	% metronidazole released from				
		Plain capsule	1cA	1cB	1cC	1cD
0.1 N HCl pH 1.2	0	0	0	0	0	0
	0.5	5.1	58.7	40.9	33.9	29.8
	1.0	90.9	67.1	53.4	40.9	40.7
	1.5	100	77.1	56.4	49.5	44.1
	2.0		87	59.3	58.1	47.4
	2.5		93.4	67.1	65.2	48.9
	3.0		100	75.1	72.2	50.73
	3.5			80.7	77	61.1
	4.0			86.6	82.1	71.6
	4.5			90.3	83.3	74.3
	5.0			94	84.5	77.3
	5.5			94	88.9	81.9
	6.0			94.2	93.7	86.6

Plain capsule: the same ingredient without polymer.

1: HPMC 15000

c; capsule dosage form

A; drug: polymer ratio 2:1   B; drug: polymer ratio 1:1

C; drug: polymer ratio 2:3   D; drug: polymer ratio 1:2

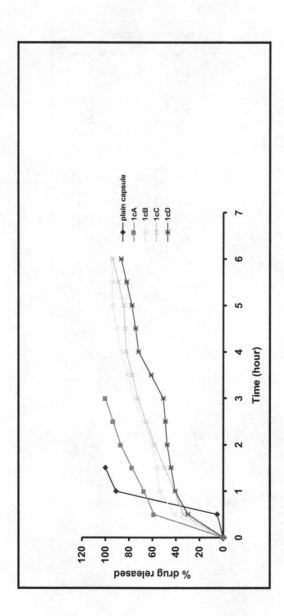

Figure (29): Release profiles of metronidazole from its capsules with different ratios of HPMC 15000, into buffer solution of pH 1.2.

Table (95): Kinetics of the dissolution data of metronidazole from its capsules prepared with different ratios of HPMC 15000 polymer.

Formula	Correlation Coefficient (r)						*Rate constant K	t½ (min)
	Zero-order	First-order	Second-order	Diffusion Model	Hixon-Crowl	Baker & Lonsdale		
Plain capsule	0.905815	-0.98376	0.870321	0.93532	0.992404	0.994495	0.00809	6.796
1cA	0.996046	-0.84467	0.662622	0.99616	0.950846	0.966908	5.35	87.19
1cB	0.976445	-0.98207	0.926569	0.988443	0.988249	0.98402	4.278	136.53
1cC	0.974601	-0.98594	0.87298	0.993916	0.99375	0.990923	4.55	120.59
1cD	0.986565	-0.96964	0.911064	0.976018	0.979706	0.963577	0.1678	297.87

* K value (dissolution rate constant) & t½ were calculated according to the order of drug release.
Plain capsule; the same ingredient without polymers.
A; Drug: polymer ratio 2:1   B; drug: polymer ratio 1:1
C; drug: polymer ratio 2:3   D; drug: polymer ratio 1:2
1; HPMC 15000   c; capsule dosage form

Table (96): In-vitro release of metronidazole from its capsules containing HPMC 4000 in different drug: polymer ratios.

Dissolution medium	Time (hour)	% metronidazole released from				
		Plain capsule	2cA	2cB	2cC	2cD
0.1 N HCl pH 1.2	0	0	0	0	0	0
	0.5	5.1	42.5	43.1	34.6	22.1
	1.0	90.9	66.6	46	45.4	37.9
	1.5	100	73.4	59.3	51.8	44.8
	2.0		80.3	72.6	58.4	51.1
	2.5		91.1	77.5	64.6	57.2
	3.0		100	82.6	72.3	63.3
	3.5			89.8	78.9	65.2
	4.0			97.1	-	67.2
	4.5			99.1	88.5	72.3
	5.0			100	92.6	77.6
	5.5				94.6	78.5
	6.0				96.5	79.5

Plain capsule: the same ingredient without polymer.

2; HPMC 4000

c; capsule dosage form

A; drug: polymer ratio 2:1   B; drug: polymer ratio 1:1

C; drug: polymer ratio 2:3   D; drug: polymer ratio 1:2

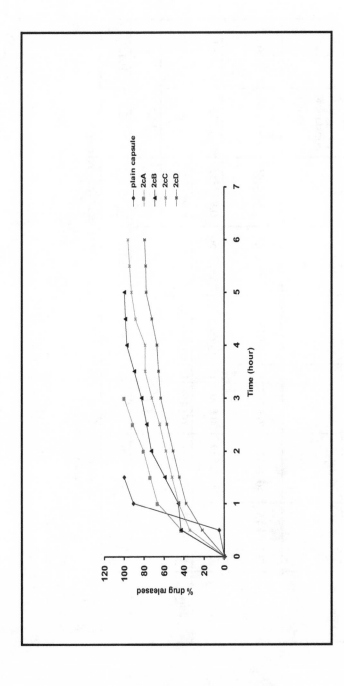

Figure (30): Release profiles of metronidazole from its capsules containing different ratios of HPMC 4000, into buffer solution of pH 1.2.

208

Table (97): Kinetics of the dissolution data of metronidazole from its capsules prepared with different ratios of polymer HPMC 4000.

Formula	Correlation Coefficient (r)						*Rate constant K	t ½ (min)
	Zero-order	First-order	Second-order	Diffusion Model	Hixon-Crowl	Baker& Lonsdale		
Plain capsule	0.905815	-0.98376	0.870321	0.93532	0.992404	0.994495	0.00809	6.796
2cA	0.973521	-0.82639	0.660151	0.988149	0.938156	0.947315	6.765	54.61
2cB	0.986552	-0.97353	0.846891	0.996438	0.992435	0.983095	4.788	109.015
2cC	0.750875	-0.87317	0.943082	0.830081	0.832906	0.85387	0.0025	3.943
2cD	0.962247	-0.99299	0.984774	0.990988	0.98725	0.995042	0.000544	101.02

* K value (dissolution rate constant) & t ½ were calculated according to the order of drug release.
Plain capsule; the same ingredient without polymers.

A; Drug: polymer ratio 2:1   B; drug: polymer ratio 1:1
C; drug: polymer ratio 2:3   D; drug: polymer ratio 1:2
2; HPMC 4000   c; capsule dosage form

Table (98): In-vitro release of metronidazole from its capsules containing
Carbopol 934 in different drug: polymer ratios.

Dissolution medium	Time (hour)	% metronidazole released from				
		Plain capsule	3cA	3cB	3cC	3cD
0.1 N HCl pH 1.2	0	0	0	0	0	0
	0.5	5.1	71.8	59.9	67.9	33.7
	1.0	90.9	91.1	87.3	89.9	57.2
	1.5	100	96.6	96.9	94.4	75.6
	2.0		100	100	97.8	94
	2.5				100	100
	3.0					
	3.5					
	4.0					
	4.5					
	5.0					
	5.5					
	6.0					

Plain capsule: the same ingredient without polymer.

3; Carbopol 934

c; capsule dosage form

A; drug: polymer ratio 2:1   B; drug: polymer ratio 1:1

C; drug: polymer ratio 2:3   D; drug: polymer ratio 1:2

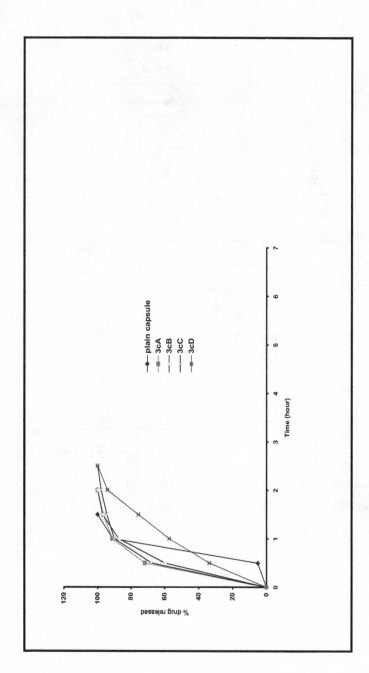

Figure (31): Release profiles of metronidazole from its capsules containing different ratios of Carbopol 934, into buffer solution of pH 1.2.

Table (99): Kinetics of the dissolution data of metronidazole from its capsules prepared with different ratios of Carbopol 934 polymer.

Formula	Correlation Coefficient (r)						*Rate constant K	t ½ (min)
	Zero-order	First-order	Second-order	Diffusion Model	Hixon-Crowl	Baker& Lonsdale		
Plain capsule	0.905815	-0.98376	0.870321	0.93532	0.992404	0.994495	0.00809	6.796
3cA	0.98325	-0.89711	0.715441	0.9954	0.979928	0.976541	10.16	24.19
3cB	0.918628	-0.96386	0.79013	0.953187	0.999207	0.994906	0.0325	29.398
3cC	0.88052	-0.94441	0.730413	0.926468	0.986388	0.981148	0.0209	45.68
3cD	0.922425	-0.94808	0.787874	0.955568	0.994221	0.993246	0.02768	34.54

* K value (dissolution rate constant) & t ½ were calculated according to the order of drug release.
Plain capsule; the same ingredient without polymers.
A; Drug: polymer ratio 2:1   B; drug: polymer ratio 1:1
C; drug: polymer ratio 2:3   D; drug: polymer ratio 1:2
3; Carbopol 934   c; capsule dosage form

Table (100): In-vitro release of metronidazole from its capsules containing sodium alginate in different drug: polymer ratios.

Dissolution medium	Time (hour)	% metronidazole released from				
		Plain capsule	4cA	4cB	4cC	4cD
0.1 N HCl pH 1.2	0	0	0	0	0	0
	0.5	5.1	7.1	4.1	6.63	6.63
	1.0	90.9	72.8	55.9	61.3	63.9
	1.5	100	84.9	67.5	77.1	82.5
	2.0		97.2	79.2	92.9	100
	2.5		99.5	79.6	99.9	
	3.0		100	80.2	100	
	3.5			81.4		
	4.0			82.5		
	4.5			84.1		
	5.0			85.7		
	5.5			86.4		
	6.0			87.2		

Plain capsule: the same ingredient without polymer.

4; sodium alginate

c; capsule dosage form

A; drug: polymer ratio 2:1   B; drug: polymer ratio 1:1

C; drug: polymer ratio 2:3   D; drug: polymer ratio 1:2

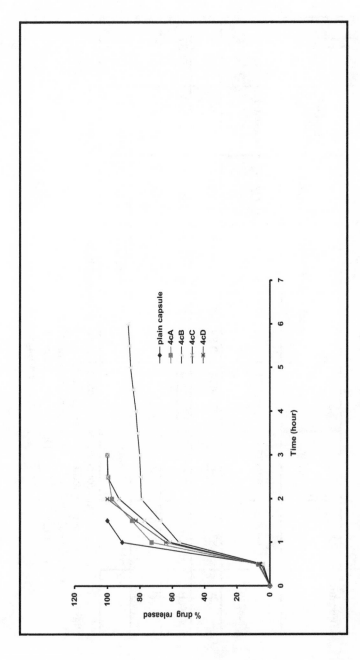

Figure (32): Release profiles of metronidazole from its capsule containing different ratios of sodium alginate, into buffer solution of pH 1.2.

Table (101): Kinetics of the dissolution data of metronidazole from its capsules prepared with different ratios of sodium alginate polymer.

Formula	Correlation Coefficient (r)						*Rate constant K	t ½ (min)
	Zero-order	First-order	Second-order	Diffusion Model	Hixon-Crowl	Baker& Lonsdale		
Plain capsule	0.905815	-0.98376	0.870321	0.93532	0.992404	0.994495	0.00809	6.796
4cA	0.83171	-0.98958	0.760072	0.891689	0.97883	0.980375	0.04561	15.19
4cB	0.726849	-0.87504	0.967069	0.813835	0.828173	0.89757	0.000184	54.37
4cC	0.727167	-0.90605	0.714285	0.962861	0.988672	0.985173	0.03201	29.86
4cD	0.950978	-0.8963	0.777001	0.975931	0.977389	0.962995	0.04308	22.19

* K value (dissolution rate constant) & t ½ were calculated according to the order of drug release.
Plain capsule; the same ingredient without polymers.

A; drug: polymer ratio 2:1   B; drug: polymer ratio 1:1
C; drug: polymer ratio 2:3   D; drug: polymer ratio 1:2
4; sodium alginate   c; capsule dosage form

215

Table (102): In-vitro release of metronidazole from its capsules containing CMC in different drug: polymer ratios.

Dissolution medium	Time (hour)	% metronidazole released from				
		Plain capsule	5cA	5cB	5cC	5cD
0.1 N HCl pH 1.2	0	0	0	0	0	0
	0.5	5.1	2.9	9.8	5.9	5.1
	1.0	90.9	61.3	51.9	49.6	48.8
	1.5	100	62.2	62.8	61.1	60.5
	2.0		75.7	73.9	72.6	72.4
	2.5		80.7	77.1	75.9	73.9
	3.0		86	80.2	79.2	75.5
	3.5		86	81.6	80.77	78.8
	4.0		86.6	83.1	82.5	82.1
	4.5		88.9	85.7	84.9	85.1
	5.0		91.3	88.2	87.4	88.2
	5.5		94.2	91.5	90.9	90.5
	6.0		97.4	95	94.4	93.1

Plain capsule: the same ingredient without polymer.

5; CMC

c; capsule dosage form

A; drug: polymer ratio 2:1   B; drug: polymer ratio 1:1

C; drug: polymer ratio 2:3   D; drug: polymer ratio 1:2

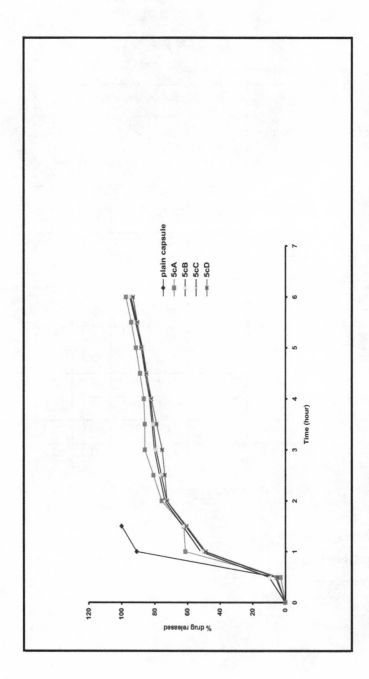

Figure (33): Release profiles of metronidazole from its capsules containing different ratios of CMC, into buffer solution of pH 1.2.

Table (103): Kinetics of the dissolution data of metronidazole from its capsules prepared with different ratios of CMC polymer.

Formula	Correlation Coefficient (r)							*Rate constant K	t ½ (min)
	Zero- order	First- order	Second - order	Diffusion Model	Hixon- Crowl	Baker& Lonsdale		
Plain capsule	0.905815	-0.98376	0.870321	0.93532	0.992404	0.994495	0.00809	6.796
5cA	0.795571	-0.96102	0.796568	0.867855	0.934868	0.973867	0.001	54.95
5cB	0.835974	-0.96774	0.869783	0.902844	0.944334	0.978785	0.00088	62.1311
5cC	0.835821	-0.9688	0.884454	0.903006	0.943536	0.980851	0.000873	62.99
5cD	0.842972	-.097656	0.934399	0.907761	0.948702	0.987289	0.000858	64.113

* K value (dissolution rate constant) & t ½ were calculated according to the order of drug release.

Plain capsule; the same ingredient without polymers.

A; Drug: polymer ratio 2:1   B; drug: polymer ratio 1:1

C; drug: polymer ratio 2:3   D; drug: polymer ratio 1:2

5; CMC   c; capsule dosage form

218

Table (104): In-vitro release of metronidazole from its capsules containing ethyl cellulose in different drug: polymer ratios.

Dissolution medium	Time (hour)	% metronidazole released from				
		Plain capsule	6cA	6cB	6cC	6cD
0.1 N HCl pH 1.2	0	0	0	0	0	0
	0.5	5.1	17.4	17.4	17.6	15.6
	1.0	90.9	58.5	57.8	54	56.8
	1.5	100	100	98.3	90.5	97.9
	2.0			100	97.6	98.3
	2.5				100	98.9
	3.0					100
	3.5					
	4.0					
	4.5					
	5.0					
	5.5					
	6.0					

Plain capsule: the same ingredient without polymer.

6; ethyl cellulose

c; capsule dosage form

A; drug: polymer ratio 2:1   B; drug: polymer ratio 1:1

C; drug: polymer ratio 2:3   D; drug: polymer ratio 1:2

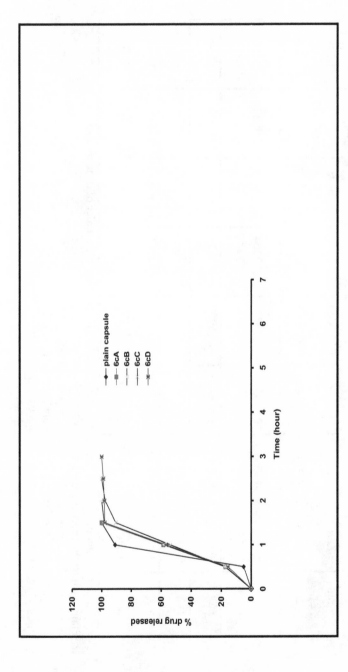

Figure (34): Release profiles of metronidazole from its capsules containing g different ratios of ethyl cellulose, into buffer solution of pH 1.2.

220

Table (105): Kinetics of the dissolution data of metronidazole from its capsules prepared with different ratios of Ethyl cellulose polymer.

Formula	Correlation Coefficient (r)						*Rate constant K	t ½ (min)
	Zero-order	First-order	Second-order	Diffusion Model	Hixon-Crowl	Baker& Lonsdale		
Plain capsule	0.905815	-0.98376	0.870321	0.93532	0.992404	0.994495	0.00809	6.796
6cA	0.99998	-0.90883	0.866545	0.996962	0.954515	0.929366	1.375	36.36
6cB	0.949548	-0.97201	0.8037	0.971142	0.977815	0.957171	0.0465	20.54
6cC	0.924771	-0.96499	0.72984	0.959467	0.994485	0.985623	0.0333	28.69
6cD	0.840978	-0.96077	0.717507	0.898412	0.91869	0.899169	0.0428	16.177

* K value (dissolution rate constant) & t ½ were calculated according to the order of drug release.
Plain capsule; the same ingredient without polymers.
A; Drug: polymer ratio 2:1 B; drug: polymer ratio 1:1
C; drug: polymer ratio 2:3 D; drug: polymer ratio 1:2
6; Ethyl cellulose   c; capsule dosage form

221

Table (106): In-vitro release of metronidazole from its capsules containing methyl cellulose in different drug: polymer ratios.

Dissolution medium	Time (hour)	% metronidazole released from				
		Plain capsule	7cA	7cB	7cC	7cD
0.1 N HCl pH 1.2	0	0	0	0	0	0
	0.5	5.1	96.6	54.8	34.5	21.3
	1.0	90.9	100	100	58.9	57.9
	1.5	100			77.7	71.2
	2.0				96.4	84.5
	2.5				99.3	95.6
	3.0				100	100
	3.5					
	4.0					
	4.5					
	5.0					
	5.5					
	6.0					

Plain capsule: the same ingredient without polymer.

7; methyl cellulose

c; capsule dosage form

A; drug: polymer ratio 2:1   B; drug: polymer ratio 1:1

C; drug: polymer ratio 2:3   D; drug: polymer ratio 1:2

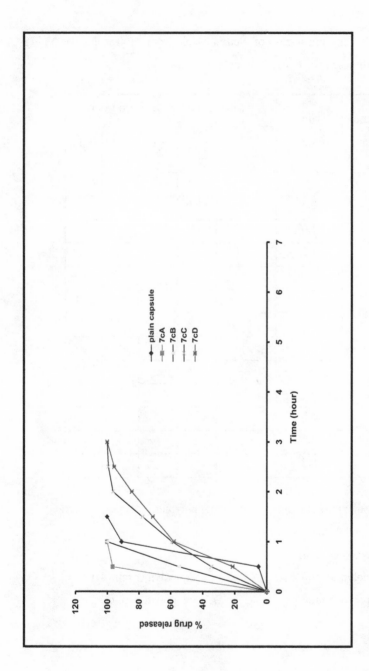

Figure (35): Release profiles of metronidazole from its capsules containing different ratios of methyl cellulose, into buffer solution of pH 1.2.

Table (107): Kinetics of the dissolution data of metronidazole from its capsules prepared with different ratios of Methyl cellulose polymer.

Formula	Correlation Coefficient (r)						*Rate constant K	t½ (min)
	Zero-order	First-order	Second-order	Diffusion Model	Hixon-Crowl	Baker& Lonsdale		
Plain capsule	0.905815	-0.98376	0.870321	0.93532	0.992404	<u>0.994495</u>	0.00809	6.796
7cA	<u>0.996196</u>	-0.92732	0.875158	0.990714	0.95608	0.974529	0.11	454.54
7cB	<u>0.98275</u>	-0.89445	0.866512	0.972482	0.925969	0.924118	1.503	33.259
7cC	0.939615	-0.97301	0.731309	0.971739	<u>0.989919</u>	0.978433	0.0255	37.46
7cD	0.95082	-0.89663	0.666918	0.980721	<u>0.986416</u>	0.98479	0.02399	39.84

* K value (dissolution rate constant) & t ½ were calculated according to the order of drug release.

Plain capsule; the same ingredient without polymers.

A; Drug: polymer ratio 2:1   B; drug: polymer ratio 1:1
C; drug: polymer ratio 2:3   D; drug: polymer ratio 1:2
7; Methyl cellulose   c; capsule dosage form

Table (108): In-vitro release of metronidazole from its capsules containing pectin in different drug: polymer ratios.

Dissolution medium	Time (hour)	% metronidazole released from				
		Plain capsule	8cA	8cB	8cC	8cD
0.1 N HCl pH 1.2	0	0	0	0	0	0
	0.5	5.1	39.2	33.4	8.8	7.9
	1.0	90.9	83.7	56.4	29.9	18.5
	1.5	100	84.1	67.5	50.9	29.1
	2.0		84.5	78.6	51.7	39
	2.5		92.7	87.8	52.5	50.7
	3.0		100	97.2	71.6	58.9
	3.5			100	90.9	67
	4.0				91.7	72.6
	4.5				92.7	78
	5.0				92.7	84.3
	5.5				97.8	93.9
	6.0				100	100

Plain capsule: the same ingredient without polymer.

c; capsule dosage form

8; pectin

A; drug: polymer ratio 2:1   B; drug: polymer ratio 1:1

C; drug: polymer ratio 2:3   D; drug: polymer ratio 1:2

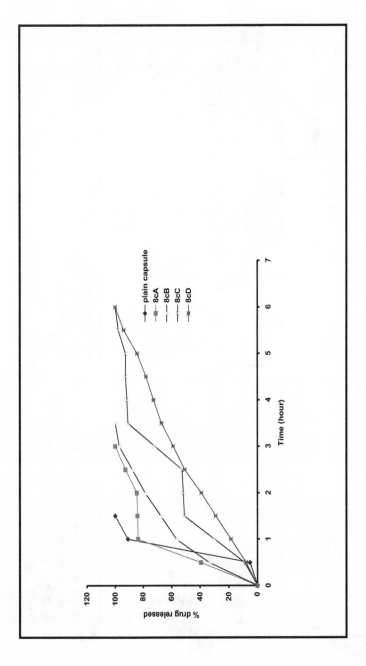

Figure (36): Release profiles of metronidazole from its capsules containing different ratios of pectin, into buffer solution of pH 1.2.

Table (109): Kinetics of the dissolution data of metronidazole from its capsules prepared with different ratios of Pectin polymer.

Formula	Correlation Coefficient (r)						*Rate constant K	t ½ (min)
	Zero-order	First-order	Second-order	Diffusion Model	Hixon-Crowl	Baker& Lonsdale		
Plain capsule	0.905815	-0.98376	0.870321	0.93532	0.992404	0.994495	0.00809	6.796
8cA	0.83007	-0.82885	0.661041	0.87768	0.91145	0.92293	0.00244	22.54
8cB	0.973896	-0.88728	0.631408	0.994327	0.980079	0.979697	7.415	45.457
8cC	0.941524	-0.8910	0.508987	0.971807	0.974664	0.96751	0.01119	85.42
8cD	0.993304	-0.78397	0.490056	0.997436	0.941298	0.91345	6.9	51.93

* K value (dissolution rate constant) & t ½ were calculated according to the order of drug release.

Plain capsule; the same ingredient without polymers.

A; drug: polymer ratio 2:1   B; drug: polymer ratio 1:1
C; drug: polymer ratio 2:3   D; drug: polymer ratio 1:2
8; Pectin   c; capsule dosage form

Table (110): In-vitro release of metronidazole from its capsules using different polymers with drug: polymer ratio 2:1.

Dissolution medium	Time (hour)	% metronidazole released from							
		1cA	2cA	3cA	4cA	5cA	6cA	7cA	8cA
0.1 N HCl pH 1.2	0	0	0	0	0	0	0	0	0
	0.5	58.7	42.5	71.8	7.1	2.9	17.4	96.6	39.2
	1.0	67.1	66.6	91.1	72.8	61.3	58.5	100	83.7
	1.5	77.1	73.4	96.6	84.9	62.2	100		84.1
	2.0	87	80.3	100	97.2	75.7			84.5
	2.5	93.4	91.1		99.5	80.7			92.7
	3.0	100	100		100	86			100
	3.5					86			
	4.0					86.6			
	4.5					88.9			
	5.0					91.3			
	5.5					94.2			
	6.0					97.4			

A; drug: polymer ratio 2:1

c; capsule dosage form

1; HPMC 15000   2; HPMC 4000   3; Carbopol 934   4; Na alginate

5; CMC   6; Ethyl cellulose   7; Methyl cellulose   8; Pectin

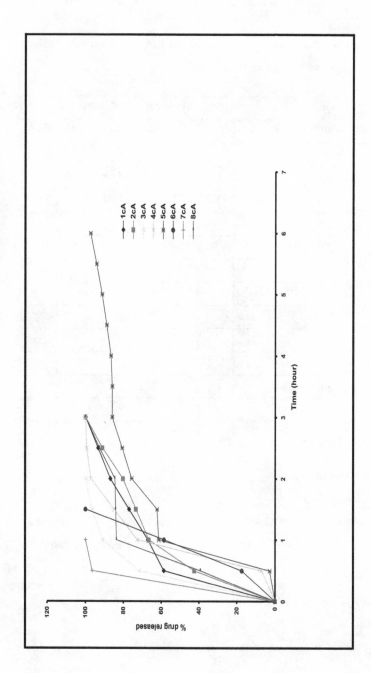

Figure (37): Release profiles of metronidazole from its capsules with different polymer in ratio 2:1, into buffer solution of pH 1.2.

Table (111): In-vitro release of metronidazole from its capsules using different polymers with drug: polymer ratio 1:1.

Dissolution medium	Time (hour)	% metronidazole released from							
		1cB	2cB	3cB	4cB	5cB	6cB	7cB	8cB
0.1 N HCl pH 1.2	0	0	0	0	0	0	0	0	0
	0.5	40.9	43.1	59.9	4.1	9.8	17.4	54.8	33.4
	1.0	53.4	46	87.3	55.9	51.9	57.8	100	56.4
	1.5	56.4	59.3	96.9	67.5	62.8	98.3		67.5
	2.0	59.3	72.6	100	79.2	73.9	100		78.6
	2.5	67.1	77.5		79.6	77.1			87.8
	3.0	75.1	82.6		80.2	80.2			97.2
	3.5	80.7	89.8		81.4	81.6			100
	4.0	86.6	97.1		82.5	83.1			
	4.5	90.3	99.1		84.1	85.7			
	5.0	94	100		85.7	88.2			
	5.5	94			86.4	91.5			
	6.0	94.2			87.2	95			

B; drug: polymer ratio 1:1

c; capsule dosage form

1; HPMC 15000 2; HPMC 4000   3; Carbopol 934   4; sodium alginate

5; CMC   6; Ethyl cellulose 7; Methyl cellulose 8; Pectin

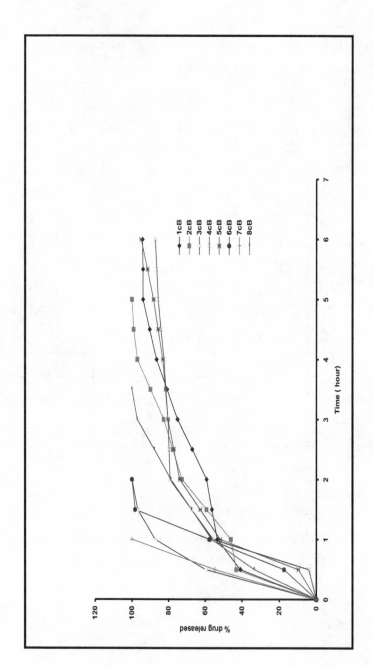

Figure (38): Release profiles of metronidazole from its capsules with different polymer in ratio1:1, into buffer solution of pH 1.2.

Table (112): In-vitro release of metronidazole from capsules using different polymers with drug: polymer ratio 2:3.

Dissolution medium	Time (hour)	% metronidazole released from							
		1cC	2cC	3cC	4cC	5cC	6cC	7cC	8cC
0.1 N HCl pH 1.2	0	0	0	0	0	0	0	0	0
	0.5	33.9	34.6	67.9	6.63	5.9	17.6	34.5	8.8
	1.0	40.9	45.4	89.9	61.3	49.6	54	58.9	29.9
	1.5	49.5	51.8	94.4	77.1	61.1	90.5	77.7	50.9
	2.0	58.1	58.4	97.8	92.9	72.6	97.6	96.4	51.7
	2.5	65.2	64.6	100	99.9	75.9	100	99.3	52.5
	3.0	72.2	72.3		100	79.2		100	71.6
	3.5	77	78.9			80.77			90.9
	4.0	82.1	78.9			82.5			91.7
	4.5	83.3	88.5			84.9			91.7
	5.0	84.5	92.6			87.4			92.7
	5.5	88.9	94.6			90.9			97.8
	6.0	93.7	96.5			94.4			100

C; drug: polymer ratio 2:3

c; capsule dosage form

1; HPMC 15000   2; HPMC 4000   3; Carbopol 934   4; sodium alginate

5; CMC   6; Ethyl cellulose   7; Methyl cellulose   8; Pectin

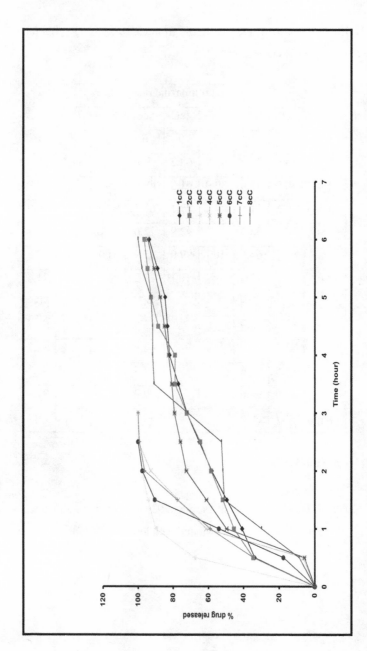

Figure (39): Release profiles of metronidazole from its capsules with different polymer in ratio 2:3, into buffer solution of pH 1.2.

233

Table (113): In-vitro release of metronidazole from capsules using different polymers with drug: polymer ratio 1:2.

Dissolution medium	Time (hour)	% metronidazole released from							
		1cD	2cD	3cD	4cD	5cD	6cD	7cD	8cD
0.1 N HCl pH 1.2	0	0	0	0	0	0	0	0	0
	0.5	29.8	22.1	33.7	6.63	5.1	15.6	21.3	7.9
	1.0	40.7	37.9	57.2	63.9	48.8	56.8	57.9	18.5
	1.5	44.1	44.8	75.6	82.5	60.5	97.9	71.2	29.1
	2.0	47.4	51.1	94	100	72.4	98.3	84.5	39
	2.5	48.9	57.2	100		73.9	98.9	95.6	50.7
	3.0	50.73	63.3			75.5	100	100	58.9
	3.5	61.1	65.2			78.8			67
	4.0	71.6	67.2			82.1			72.6
	4.5	74.3	72.3			85.1			78
	5.0	77.3	77.6			88.2			84.3
	5.5	81.9	78.5			90.5			93.9
	6.0	86.6	79.5			93.1			100

D; drug: polymer ratio 1:2

c; capsule dosage form

1; HPMC 15000 2; HPMC 4000   3; Carbopol 934   4; sodium alginate

5; CMC   6; Ethyl cellulose   7; Methyl cellulose   8; Pectin

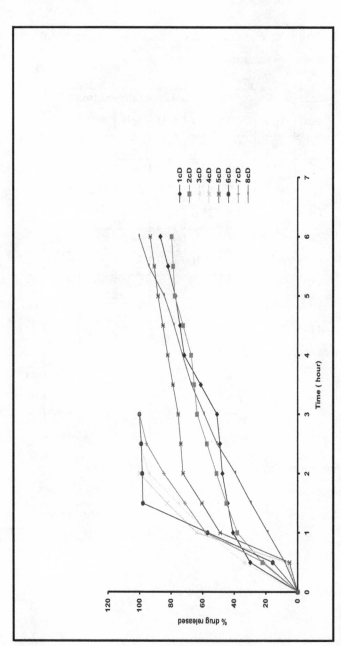

Figure (40): Release profiles of metronidazole from its capsules with different polymer in ratio 1:2, into buffer solution of pH 1.2.

Table (114): Floating behavior of metronidazole capsules using HPMC 15000 in different drug: polymer ratios.

Behavior	1cA	1cB	1cC	1cD	Plain capsule
Buoyancy lag time (minutes)	Zero	Zero	Zero	Zero	Zero
Buoyancy duration (minutes)	25	150	360	360	17

Table (115): Floating behavior of metronidazole capsules using HPMC 4000 in different drug: polymer ratios.

Behavior	2cA	2cB	2cC	2cD	Plain capsule
Buoyancy lag time (minutes)	Zero	Zero	Zero	Zero	Zero
Buoyancy duration (minutes)	20	20	258	360	17

Table (116): Floating behavior of metronidazole capsules using Carbopol 934 in different drug: polymer ratios.

Behavior	3cA	3cB	3cC	3cD	Plain capsule
Buoyancy lag time (minutes)	Zero	Zero	Zero	Zero	Zero
Buoyancy duration (minutes)	20	35	20	20	17

Table (117): Floating behavior of metronidazole capsules using sodium alginate in different drug: polymer ratios.

Behavior	4cA	4cB	4cC	4cD	Plain capsule
Buoyancy lag time (minutes)	Zero	Zero	Zero	Zero	Zero
Buoyancy duration (minutes)	20	20	17	17	17

Table (118): Floating behavior of metronidazole capsules containing CMC in different drug: polymer ratios.

Behavior	5cA	5cB	5cC	5cD	Plain capsule
Buoyancy lag time (minutes)	Zero	Zero	Zero	Zero	Zero
Buoyancy duration (minutes)	20	20	20	20	17

Table (119): Floating behavior of metronidazole capsules using ethyl cellulose in different drug: polymer ratios.

Behavior	6cA	6cB	6cC	6cD	Plain capsule
Buoyancy lag time (minutes)	Zero	Zero	Zero	Zero	Zero
Buoyancy duration (minutes)	20	20	20	30	17

Table (120): Floating behavior of metronidazole capsules using methyl cellulose in different drug: polymer ratios.

Behavior	7cA	7cB	7cC	7cD	Plain capsule
Buoyancy lag time (minutes)	Zero	Zero	Zero	Zero	Zero
Buoyancy duration (minutes)	21	30	66	72	17

Table (121): Floating behavior of metronidazole capsules using pectin in different drug: polymer ratios.

Behavior	8cA	8cB	8cC	8cD	Plain capsule
Buoyancy lag time (minutes)	Zero	Zero	Zero	Zero	Zero
Buoyancy duration (minutes)	20	20	20	360	17

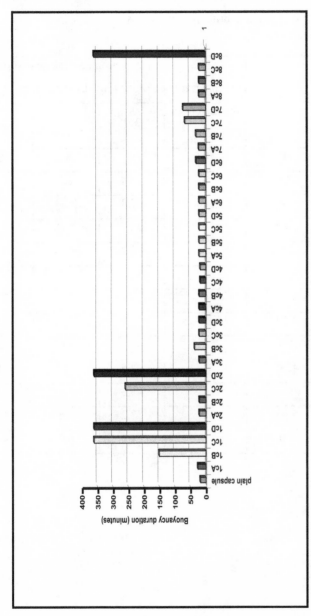

Figure (41): Histogram showing the buoyancy duration of different metronidazole floating capsules formulae.

c; capsule dosage form.

A, B, C, D; drug: polymer ratios 2:1, 1:1, 2:3, 1:2, respectively.

1,2,3,4,5,6,7,8 polymers HPMC 15000, HPMC 4000, Carbopol 934, sodium alginate, CMC, ethyl cellulose, methyl cellulose, and pectin , respectively.

240

Table (122): In-vitro release of metronidazole from its floating microspheres with Eudragit S 100 in different drug: polymer ratios.

Dissolution medium	Time (hour)	% metronidazole released from Plain drug	% metronidazole released from following drug: polymer ratios		
			2: 1	1:1	1:2
0.1 N HCl pH 1.2	0	0	0	0	0
	0.5	40	17.4	2.3	1.5
	1.0	100	27.3	2.34	1.7
	1.30		28.7	2.41	1.9
	2.0		30.2	2.44	2.1
	2.30		31.8	2.48	2.19
	3.0		33.4	2.5	2.2
	3.30		37.7	2.7	2.2
	4.0		42.1	2.8	2.3
	4.30		42.5	4	3
	5.0		45.5	4.9	3.3
	5.30		57.2	5.8	4
	6.0		69.1	6.9	4.1

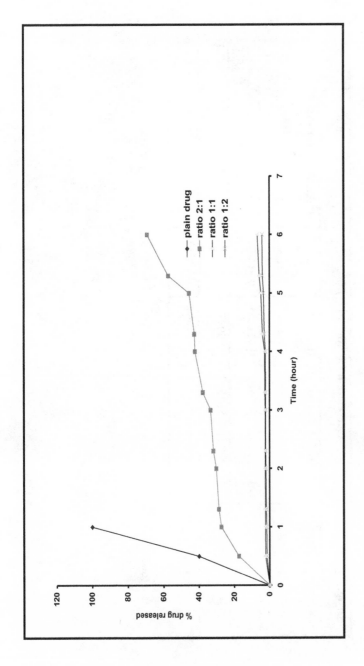

Figure (42): Release profiles of metronidazole floating microspheres prepared with different ratios of Eudragit S100, into buffer solution of pH 1.2.

242

Table (123): Kinetics of the dissolution data of metronidazole from its microspheres prepared with different ratios of Eudragit S100 polymer.

Drug: polymer ratio	Correlation Coefficient (r)						*Rate constant K	t ½ (min)
	Zero - order	First- order	Second- order	Diffusion Model	Hixon- Crowl	Baker& Lonsdale		
2:1	0.944111	-0.89524	0.827869	0.911865	0.914075	0.845202	0.1226	407.75
1:1	0.865106	-0.86347	0.861817	0.790975	0.86402	0.821624	0.0126	3967.447
1:2	0.935978	-0.93505	0.934112	0.891609	0.93536	0.897363	0.00745	6710.465

* K value (dissolution rate constant) & t ½ were calculated according to the order of drug release.

Table (124): The percent yield, the percent microspheres floating after 6 hours, and microspheres loading efficiency of different prepared floating microspheres of metronidazole.

Polymer	Drug: polymer ratio	Yield %	%of microspheres floating after 6 hours	Loading efficiency %
Eudragit S100	2:1	54.3	85%	22.8
	1:1	43	92%	29.5
	1:2	59.6	91%	22.1

Table (125): The particle size distribution for different formulae of metronidazole microspheres prepared with Eudragit S100.

Drug: polymer ratio	% weight retained in the following sieve size range (um)				
	1000-800	800-450	450-250	250-90	90-0
2:1	2	5.4	4.41	30.4	57.7
1:1	2.5	6.3	10.11	46.28	34.81
1:2	2.6	8	20	53.6	15.8

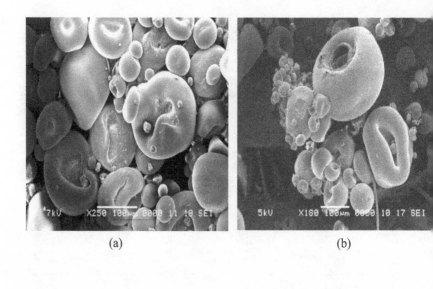

(a)　　　　　　　　　　　　　　　　(b)

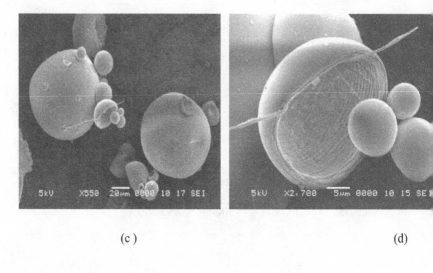

(c)　　　　　　　　　　　　　　　　(d)

Figure (43): Scanning electron micrographs of metronidazole microballoons
containing Eudragit S100 in drug: polymer ratio 2:1.(a), (b), (c) round structure o
prepared microballoons; (d) internal view of microballoon.

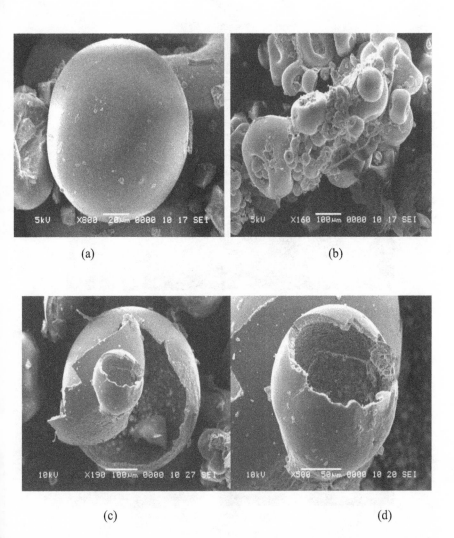

(a)   (b)

(c)   (d)

Figure (44): Scanning electron micrographs. (a), and (b) microspheres containing metronidazole: Eudragit S100 drug: polymer ratio 1:1; (c) and (d) internal view.

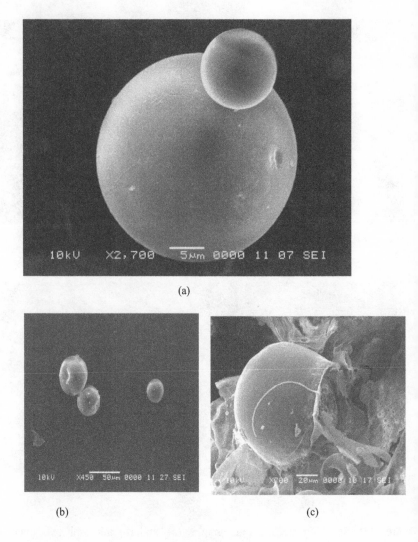

(a)

(b)   (c)

Figure (45): Scanning electron micrographs. (a), and (b) metronidazole microspheres containing Eudragit S100 in drug: polymer ratio 1:2; (c) internal view.

Results and Discussion

Metronidazole was formulated in floating capsules and floating microspheres (microballoons) using different polymers in order to retard the in-vitro release and hence to sustain the in-vivo bioavailability as will as to increase the gastric residence time of metronidazole. The target of controlling the dissolution of metronidazole in the stomach is to exert its local effect for eradication of Helicobacter pylori organism which found to be responsible for peptic ulcer disease. Non effervescent floating system technique was performed in this study using gel forming polymer metronidazole capsules dosage forms and using solvent-diffusion and evaporation method for metronidazole microspheres (microballoons).

Table (76) showed the bulk density of metronidazole, polymers, diluents, and additives that were chosen for formulation of metronidazole floating capsules.

Tables (78-85) represent the different formulae of metronidazole capsule prepared using different drug: polymer ratios of the selected polymers; HPMC 15000, HPMC 4000, Carbopol 934, sodium alginate, CMC, ethyl cellulose, methyl cellulose, and pectin. The Tables showed each ingredients weight and the corresponding volume. It is clear that the bulk density of each formula will be less than 1 gm/cm^3. Formulation process was tried by using avicel and aerosil as diluent and lubricant, respectively.

The chosen polymers were selected so that they can absorb a significant amount of water while maintaining a distinct three dimensional

248

structure. As a result, they conform to the definition of hydrogels and be able to form an outer gel layer after the dissolution of the gelatin capsule in the gastric juice (Gerogiannis et al., 1993). Dissolution or degradation then occurs to the formed gel layer by the process of erosion and a creation of new gel layers takes place (Gehvrke and Lee, 1990). In the same time, water uptake and consequently, weight gain, should be compensated by adequate swelling in order to keep the dosage form at buoyant state (Gerogiannis et al., 1993).

Formulation of a floating dosage form requires a nondigestable hydrophilic polymer that can absorb a significant amount of water to form a gel in situ. Drug release is controlled by penetration of water through the gel layer produced by hydration of the polymer and diffusion of the drug through the swollen, hydrated matrix in addition to erosion of the gelled layer. Higher molecular weight polymers and slower rates of polymer hydration are usually followed by enhanced floating behavior (Lordi, 1986 and Gerogiannis et al., 1993). Low molecular weight polymers release drug largely by attrition, since a significant intact hydrated layers is not maintained. The extent to which diffusion or erosion controls the release depends on the polymer selected as well as the drug: polymer ratio. Polymers such as HPMC high viscosity, hydroxypropylcellulose (HPC) grade H and polyethylene oxide (poly ox) grades WSR-303 were reported to have enhanced floating behaviors beside their retarding properties (Lordi, 1986 and Gerogiannis et al., 1993).

Tables (86-93) illustrate the evaluation of metronidazole content in its capsule dosage forms prepared with different ratios of the selected polymers.

It is clear that, the average drug content ranged from 92.6 % to 102.4 % with standard deviation ranges from   0.8 to 3.96. Also, it is clear that the lowest coefficient of variation was 0.8 %   concerning formula 1cB which contain polymer HPMC 15000 in drug: polymer ratio 1:1, while metronidazole capsule containing polymer CMC (formula 5cD)   with drug: polymer ratio 1:2 showed the highest coefficient of variation of the drug content. Figure (28) showed a histogram of drug content of metronidazole capsule formulae.

a- In-vitro release and floating properties of metronidazole capsule dosage form

1-Formulae containing HPMC 15000

Table (94) and Figure (29) show metronidazole release from 1cA, 1cB, 1cC, and1cD formulae that contain drug: polymer ratios 2:1, 1:1, 2:3, and 1:2, respectively, compared with plain capsule (capsules that devoid of any polymer).The release study was carried out in simulated gastric fluid of pH 1.2 for 6 hours. Formula 1cD which contain drug: polymer ratio 1:2 showed the minimum in-vitro release (86.6 %) after 6 hours of dissolution. In contrast, formula 1cA that contain drug: polymer ratio 2:1 showed the maximum in-vitro release of drug content (100 %) after 3 hours of dissolution.

The investigated formulae containing metronidazole and HPMC 15000 in different drug: polymer ratios can be arranged, in ascending manner, regarding the in-vitro release of metronidazole within 6 hours dissolution, as follows: formula containing drug: polymer ratio 1:2 (1cD),

250

formula containing drug: polymer ratio 2:3 (1cC), formula containing drug: polymer ratio 1:1 (1cB), then finally formula containing drug: polymer ratio 2:1 (1cA).

Data in Table (95) illustrate the kinetic treatment and parameters for the in-vitro release of metronidazole from its capsule dosage form. It is clear that, Higuchi-model of diffusion controlled the release of drug from formulae 1cA, 1cB, and 1cC with t ½ values of 87.19, 136.53, and 120.59 min, respectively.

Table (114) shows the floating properties of the four formulae on a simulated gastric fluid. Floating time was of a short value (25 minutes) concerning formula1cA (drug: polymer ratio 2:1) while was of a medium value (150 minutes) in case of formula 1cB (drug: polymer ratio 1:1).Whereas formula 1cC (drug: polymer ratio 2:3) and formula 1cD (drug: polymer ratio 1:2) succeed to float all the dissolution time of 6 hours.

2-Formulae containing HPMC 4000

Table (96) and Figure (30) show metronidazole release from 2cA, 2cB, 2cC, and 2cD formulae that contain drug: polymer ratios 2:1, 1:1, 2:3, and 1:2, respectively, in addition to the release of the drug from the plain capsule (capsules that devoid of any polymer).The release study was carried out in simulated gastric fluid of pH 1.2 for 6 hours. The minimum in-vitro release was 79.5 % after 6 hours dissolution concerning formula 2cD which contain drug: polymer ratio 1:2. On the contrary, the maximum in-vitro release of drug content was 100 % after 3 hours dissolution from formula 2cA that contain drug: polymer ratio 2:1.

251

The investigated capsule formulae containing metronidazole and HPMC 4000 in different drug: polymer ratios can be arranged, in ascending order, concerning the in-vitro release of metronidazole within 6 hours dissolution, as follow: formula containing drug: polymer ratio 1:2 (2cD), formula containing drug: polymer ratio 2:3 (2cC), formula containing drug: polymer ratio 1:1 (2cB), then formula containing drug: polymer ratio 2:1 (2cA).

Data in Table (97) shows the kinetic treatment for the in-vitro release of metronidazole from its capsule dosage form prepared with HPMC 4000 with various drug: polymer ratios. It can be observed that, the formulae 2cA (drug: polymer ratio 2:1) and formula 2cB (drug: polymer ratio 1:1) followed Higuchi-model of diffusion with t ½ values of 54.6, and 109.015 min, respectively. While for metronidazole capsules containing HPMC 4000 with drug: polymer ratio 2:3 (formula 2cC) obeys second order kinetic with t ½value of 3.943 minutes. Finally, the order of release of formula 2cD (drug: polymer ratio 1:2) was observed to follow Baker and Lansdale equation with t ½ value of 101.02 min.

Table (115) shows the floating properties of the four formulae on a simulated gastric fluid. The floating time found to be 20 minutes for both formulae 2cA (drug: polymer ratio 2:1) and 2cB (drug: polymer ratio 1:1), while formula 2cC (drug: polymer ratio 2:3) shows much longer floating time which equal to 258 minutes, finally formula 2cD (drug: polymer ratio 1:2) success to float on the dissolution medium for all the 6 hours dissolution time.

252

3-Formulae containing Carbopol 934

Table (98) and Figure (31) shows metronidazole release from 3cA, 3cB, 3cC, and 3cD formulae that contain drug: polymer ratios 2:1, 1:1, 2:3, and 1:2, respectively, compared with plain capsule (capsules that devoid of any polymer).The release study was carried out in simulated gastric fluid of pH 1.2 for 6 hours. It is clear that those formulae prepared with Carbopol 934 in different drug: polymer ratios showed rapid release of their drug content since with formula 3cA(drug; polymer ratio 2:1) and formula 3cB (drug: polymer ratio 1:1) reach the maximum release of their drug content 100% after 2 hours of dissolution .While formula 3cC (drug: polymer ratio 2:3) and formula 3cD (drug: polymer ratio 1:2) reach the maximum release of their drug content 100 % after 2.5 hours of dissolution study.

Data in Table (99) shows the kinetic treatment for the in-vitro release of metronidazole from its capsule dosage form prepared with Carbopol 934 with various drug: polymer ratios. It is obvious that the dissolution rate of metronidazole capsules containing Carbopol 934 in drug: polymer ratio 1:1 (formula 3cB), drug: polymer ratio 2:3 (formula 3cC), and drug: polymer ratio 1:2 (formula 3cD) follows Hixson-Crowell model with t ½ values of 29.398, 45.68, and 34.54 minutes, respectively. Concerning the dissolution of metronidazole capsules that prepared with Carbopol 934 with drug: polymer ratio 2:1 (formula 3cA) follows Higuchi-Diffusion model with t ½ value of 24.19 minutes.

Table (116) shows the floating properties of the four formulae 3cA, 3cB, 3cC, and 3cD on a simulated gastric fluid which ranged from 20 to 35 minutes.

4-Formulae containing sodium alginate

Table (100) and Figure (32) represent metronidazole release from 4cA, 4cB, 4cC, and 4cD formulae that contain drug: polymer ratios 2:1, 1:1, 2:3, and 1:2, respectively, in addition to their release from plain capsule (capsules that devoid of any polymer).The release study was carried out in simulated gastric fluid of pH 1.2 for 6 hours. The minimum in-vitro release was 87.2 % after 6 hours dissolution concerning formula 4cB which contain sodium alginate in drug: polymer ratio 1:1. On the contrary, the maximum in-vitro release of drug content was 100 % after 2 hours dissolution from formula 4cD that contain sodium alginate in drug: polymer ratio 1:2.

The investigated capsule formulae containing metronidazole and sodium alginate in different drug: polymer ratios can be arranged, in ascending way, concerning the in-vitro release of metronidazole during 6 hours dissolution, as follow: capsules containing drug: polymer ratio 2:3 (formula 4cB), capsules containing drug: polymer ratio 2:1 (formula 4cA), capsules containing drug: polymer ratio 2:3 (formula 4cC), then capsules containing drug: polymer ratio 1:2 (formula 4cD).

Data in Table (101) shows the kinetic treatment for the in-vitro release of metronidazole from its capsules dosage form prepared with sodium alginate with various drug: polymer ratios. It is clear that, the order of release of formula 4cC (drug: polymer ratio 2:3) and formula 4cD (drug: polymer ratio 1:2) obeys Hixson-Crowell model with t½ values of 29.86, and 22.19 minutes, respectively. While for formula 4cA (drug: polymer ratio 2:1) follows first order kinetic with t ½ value of 15.19 minutes. Finally,

254

formula 4cB which contain drug: polymer ratio 2:3 exhibits second order release with t ½ value of 54.37 minutes.

Table (117) shows the floating properties of the four formulae 4cA, 4cB, 4cC, and 4cD on a simulated gastric fluid. It is clear that the floating time of the four formulae prepared with sodium alginate has no significant difference and ranged from 17 to 20 minutes.

5-Formulae containing CMC

Table (102) and Figure (33) shows metronidazole release from 5cA, 5cB, 5cC, and 5cD formulae that contain drug: polymer ratios 2:1, 1:1, 2:3, and 1:2, respectively, compared with plain capsule (capsules that devoid of any polymer).The release study was carried out in simulated gastric fluid of pH 1.2 for 6 hours. The minimum in-vitro release was 93.1% after 6 hours dissolution concerning formula 5cD which contain CMC in drug: polymer ratio 1:2. While, the maximum in-vitro release of drug content was 97.4 % after 6 hours from formula 5cA that contain drug: polymer ratio 2:1.

The investigated capsule formulae containing metronidazole and CMC in different drug: polymer ratios can be arranged, in ascending way, concerning the in-vitro release of metronidazole within 6 hours dissolution, as follow: formula containing drug: polymer ratio 1:2 (5cD), formula containing drug: polymer ratio 2:3 (5cC), formula containing drug: polymer ratio 1:1 (5cB), then formula containing drug: polymer ratio 2:1 (5cA).

255

Data in Table (103) shows the kinetic treatment for the in-vitro release of metronidazole from its capsules dosage form prepared with CMC with various drug: polymer ratios. It can be observed that, the Baker and Lansdale equation controlled the release of metronidazole from all the prepared formulae 5cA, 5cB, 5cC, and 5cD with t ½ values of 54.95, 62.13, 62.99, and 64.113 minutes, respectively.

Table (118) shows the floating properties of the four formulae on a simulated gastric fluid. The floating time was found to be 20 minutes for all the prepared four formulae 5cA, 5cB, 5cC, and 5cD. It is clear that this time that considered necessary for capsules to rupture. All prepared formulae show no floating properties on the dissolution medium so their contents sink immediately.

6-Formulae containing ethyl cellulose

Table (104) and Figure (34) represent metronidazole release from 6cA, 6cB, 6cC, and 6cD formulae that contain ethyl cellulose with drug: polymer ratios 2:1, 1:1, 2:3, and 1:2, respectively, compared with plain capsule (capsules that devoid of any polymer).The release study was carried out in simulated gastric fluid of pH 1.2 for 6 hours. It is obvious that all formulae showed a rapid release of their content of metronidazole as shown with formula 6cA (drug: polymer ratio 2:1) which reach the maximum release of 100% after only 1.5 hours ,while formula 6cD that contain ethyl cellulose in drug: polymer ratio 1:2 reach maximum release of 100 % after 3 hours.

The investigated capsule formulae containing metronidazole and ethyl cellulose in different drug: polymer ratios can be arranged, in ascending way, concerning the in-vitro release of metronidazole within 6 hours dissolution, as follow: formula containing drug: polymer ratio 1:2 (6cD), formula containing drug: polymer ratio 2:3 (6cC), formula containing drug: polymer ratio 1:1 (6cB), then finally, formula containing drug: polymer ratio 2:1 (6cA).

Data in Table (105) shows the kinetic treatment and parameters for the in-vitro release of metronidazole from its capsule dosage form prepared with ethyl cellulose with various drug: polymer ratios. It can be observed that, the formula 6cB (drug: polymer ratio 1:1) and formula 6cC (drug: polymer ratio 2:3), and formula 6cd (drug: polymer ratio 1:2) obey Hixson-Crowell model with t ½ values of 20.54, 28.69, and 16.177 minutes, respectively. Concerning formula 6vA (drug: polymer ratio 2:1) follows zero order kinetic with t ½ value of 36.36 minutes.

Table (119) shows the floating properties of the four formulae on a simulated gastric fluid. The floating time found to range from 20 to 30 minutes for all the prepared four formulae 6cA, 6cB, 6cC, and 6cD. It is clear that this time that considered necessary for capsules to rupture. All prepared formulae show no floating properties on the dissolution medium so their contents sink immediately.

7-Formulae containing methyl cellulose

Table (106) and Figure (35) represent metronidazole release from 7cA, 7cB, 7cC, and 7cD formulae that contain methyl cellulose with drug:

257

polymer ratios 2:1, 1:1, 2:3, and 1:2, respectively, in addition to the release of the drug from plain capsule (capsules that devoid of any polymer).The release study was carried out in simulated gastric fluid of pH 1.2 for 6 hours. It is obvious that all formulae showed a rapid release of their content of metronidazole as shown with formulae 7cA (drug: polymer ratio 2:1) and formula 7cB (drug: polymer ratio 1:1) which reach the maximum release of 100% after only one hour, while formula 7cC that contain methyl cellulose in drug: polymer ratio 2:3 and formula 7cD which contain methyl cellulose in drug: polymer ratio 1:2 reach maximum release of 100 % after 3 hours.

Data in Table (107) shows the kinetic treatment for the in-vitro release data of metronidazole from its capsule dosage form prepared with methyl cellulose with various drug: polymer ratios. It can be observed that, the formula 7cC (drug: polymer ratio 2:3) and formula 7cD (drug: polymer ratio 1:2) follow Hixson-Crowell model with t ½ values of 37.46, and 39.84 minutes, respectively.

Table (120) shows the floating properties of the four formulae on a simulated gastric fluid. The investigated capsules formulae containing metronidazole with different ratios of methyl cellulose can be arranged, in ascending manner, according to the floating time on the dissolution medium, as follows: formula 7cA (drug: polymer ratio 2:1), formula 7cB (drug: polymer ratio 1:1), formula 7cC(drug: polymer ratio 2:3), finally, formula 7cD(drug: polymer ratio 1:2).

<u>8-Formulae containing pectin</u>

Table (108) and Figure (36) represent metronidazole release from 8cA, 8cB, 8cC, and 8cD formulae that contain pectin with drug: polymer ratios 2:1, 1:1, 2:3, and 1:2, respectively, compared with plain capsule (capsules that devoid of any polymer).The release study was carried in simulated gastric fluid of pH 1.2. All the prepared formulae with different ratios of pectin found to reach the maximum release of their drug content (100%) during 6 hours dissolution.

The investigated capsule formulae containing metronidazole and pectin in different drug: polymer ratios can be arranged, in ascending way, concerning the in-vitro release of metronidazole within 6 hours dissolution, as follow: formula containing drug: polymer ratio 2:3 (8cC), and formula containing drug: polymer ratio 1:2 (8cD), formula containing drug: polymer ratio 1:1 (8cB), and finally formula containing drug: polymer ratio 2:1 (8cA).

Data in Table (109) showed the kinetic treatment for the in-vitro release data of metronidazole from its capsule dosage form prepared with pectin with various drug: polymer ratios. It can be observed that, both formulae 8cB (drug: polymer ratio 1:1) and formula 8cD (drug: polymer ratio 1:2) was found to obey Higuchi-Diffusion model with t ½ values of 45.457, and 51.93 minutes, respectively. Concerning formula 8cA (drug: polymer ratio 2:1) was found to follow Baker and Lansdale equation with t ½ value of 22.54 minutes. Regarding formula 8cC (drug: polymer 2:3) was follows Hixson-Crowell model with t ½ 85.42 minutes.

Table (121) shows the floating properties of the four the formulae on a simulated gastric fluid. The floating time was found to be the same for the formulae 8cA, 8cB, and 8cC with value of 20 minutes. Floatation time of 6 hours was achieved with formula 8cD (drug: polymer ratio 1:2).

The release of metronidazole from plain capsules (capsules that contain the same ingredients of other formulae without any polymers) was compared with the other formulae. It is clear that, the entire drug content of plain capsules was released after 1.5 hours .This finding comply with the USP (2000) requirements which stated that not less than 85% of the labeled amount of metronidazole to be dissolved in one hour.

From the kinetic treatment of the in-vitro release data of metronidazole from its plain capsules, it can be observed that the order of release from the plain capsules obeys Baker and Lonsdale equation with t ½ value of 6.796 minutes.

It is clear that, the plain capsule have no significant floating properties as it float for only 17 minutes on the dissolution medium, then the capsules rupture and their content fall down.

The in-vitro release of metronidazole from different formulated capsules using the selected polymers with the same drug: polymer ratio 2:1 is shown in Table (110) and illustrated in Figure (37).The maximum retardation time of drug release was 6 hours from formula 5cA containing CMC which release 97.4% metronidazole from its capsules. The retardation of metronidazole release from capsules was arranged, in ascending order, as follow: CMC (formula 5cA) >HPMC 15000 (formula 1cA), HPMC 4000 (formula 2cA), sodium alginate (formula 4cA), and pectin (formula 8cA) > methyl cellulose (formula 7tA).

Table (111) and Figure (38) demonstrates metronidazole release profiles from metronidazole capsules prepared with the selected polymers in drug: polymer ratio 1:1. The minimum in-vitro release was 87.2% after 6 hours dissolution concerning formula 4cB (containing Na alginate). The retardation of metronidazole capsules was arranged, in ascending manner, as follows: sodium alginate (formula 4cB) >HPMC 15000 (formula 1cB) > CMC (formula 5cB) > HPMC 4000 (formula 2cB) >pectin (formula 8cB) > Carbopol 934 (formula 3cB) & ethyl cellulose (formula 6cB) > methyl cellulose (formula 7cB).

Table (112) and Figure (39) demonstrates metronidazole release profiles from metronidazole capsules prepared with the selected polymers in drug: polymer ratio 2:3. The maximum retardation of release was 93.7% after 6 hours dissolution concerning formula 1cC (containing HPMC 15000). The retardation of metronidazole capsules was arranged, in ascending manner, as follows: HPMC 15000 (formula 1cC) > CMC (formula 5cC) > HPMC 4000 (formula 2cC) > pectin (formula 8cC) > sodium alginate (formula 4cC) &methyl cellulose (formula 7cC) >Carbopol 934 (formula 3cC) & ethyl cellulose (formula 6cC).

Table (113) and Figure (40) demonstrates metronidazole release profiles from metronidazole capsules prepared with the selected polymers in drug: polymer ratio 1:2. The maximum retardation of release was 79.5%

after 6 hours dissolution concerning formula 2cD (containing HPMC 4000). The retardation of metronidazole capsules was arranged, in ascending manner, as follows: HPMC 4000 (formula 2cD) > HPMC 15000 (formula 1cD) > CMC (formula 5cD) > pectin (formula 8cD) > ethyl cellulose (formula 6cD) & methyl cellulose (formula 7cD) > Carbopol 934 (formula 3cD) > sodium alginate (formula 4cD).

Figure (41) illustrated a histogram that explains the buoyancy duration of the prepared capsule formulae of metronidazole using different polymers with various drug: polymer ratios. It is clear that, only those formulae containing pectin in drug: polymer ratio 1:2 (formula 8cD), HPMC 15000 in drug: polymer ratios 1:2 (formula 1cD) and 2:3 (formula 1cC), and finally HPMC 4000 in drug: polymer ratio 1:2 (formula 2cD) be able to float for all dissolution time while the rest of formulae have floating time ranged from 17 to 258 minutes.

b- In vitro release and floating properties of metronidazole microspheres (microballoons):

The key factor for preparing microballoons having a smooth outer surface and low density are the formation of an o/w emulsion at the initial stage and the precipitation of polymer on the surface of the dispersed droplet. To perform these requirements, the combination of an acrylic resin polymer, Eudragit S, and a mixed solvent of ethanol and dichloromethane was chosen (Kawashima et al., 1991, 1992). Ethanol and dichloromethane are good and poor solvents for Eudragit S, respectively. The microspheres were generated by an emulsion solvent-diffusion and evaporation method, Figure (46).

262

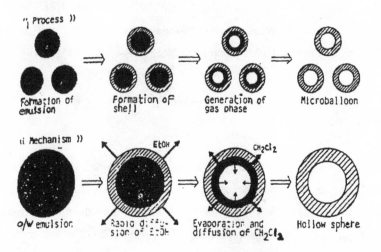

Figure (46): Preparation procedure and mechanism of microballoons formation by the emulsion-solvent diffusion method (Kumaresh etal., 2001).

As ethanol, a good solvent for the acrylic polymer preferentially diffuses out of dispersed droplet (organic phase) into an aqueous phase, the acrylic polymer instantly solidifies as a thin film at the interface between the aqueous phase and the organic phase. As ethanol quickly diffused out of the organic phase (polymer solution) into the aqueous phase, Eudragit S100 dissolved in ethanol and solidified in fiber-like aggregate. Kawashima et al., 1993 reported that when the diffusion rate of solvent out of emulsion droplet was too slow, microspheres coalesced together. Conversely, when the diffusion rate of solvent is too fast, the solvent may diffuse into the aqueous phase before stable emulsion droplet are developed, causing the aggregation of embryonic microspheres droplets. However, when a mixture of ethanol, isopropanol, and dichloromethane was used together, the yield was

263

improved significantly, indicating an optimum diffusion rate of the solvent .Since the diffusion rate of isopropanol into the aqueous phase is slower than that of ethanol, so the addition of isopropanol to the organic mixture provide more time for the droplet formation and improve the microspheres yield. The optimal results based on the yield of microspheres, were obtained when the ratio of ethanol: isopropanol: dichloromethane was 8: 2: 5.

The physico-chemical properties of the drug were also affecting the loading efficiency into the acrylic floating microspheres. When the drug is soluble in alcohol (ethanol and isopropanol), it is possible that the drug may diffuse out of emulsion droplets together with alcohol before the droplet solidification, leading to a low loading efficiency. This escaping tendency of the drug would become prominent when the solubility of the drug in dichloromethane is low, since the drug will preferentially partition into the alcohol phase when it moves into the aqueous phase from a mixture with dichloromethane. This is supported from the results shown in Table (124) of loading efficiency of metronidazole, which have relatively lower solubility in dichloromethane. So the unsatisfactory loading efficiency of metronidazole into acrylic floating microspheres was attributed to its high solubility in both alcohol and in water and low solubility in dichloromethane, which warrants the highest escaping tendency.

The high surface tension of water caused the solidification and aggregation of the acrylic polymer (Eudragit S100) on the surface of the aqueous phase. To minimize the contact of polymer solution with the air-water interface and develop a continuous process for preparing microspheres, the polymer solution was introduced into the aqueous phase

264

by a syringe without contacting the surface of the water. This method improved the yield of microspheres and reduced the extent of aggregate formation and made it possible to make microspheres continuously.

The speed of propeller rotation was adjusted at 250 rpm. It was found by Lee et al., 1999 that below 250 rpm the shear force will not be sufficient to form stable emulsion droplets. Larger droplets will be consequently formed and they will aggregate eventually. On the other hand at above 250 rpm the average particle size together with the loading efficiency will decreased.

The temperature of the dispersing medium was also an important factor in the formation of microspheres, because it controls the evaporation rate of the solvents. The temperature of the dispersing medium was adjusted at 25-28°C, which is reported to be the optimum temperature to form good microspheres (Lee et al., 1999). At lower temperatures (10°C); prepared microspheres had crushed and irregularly shaped morphology. The shell of microspheres was translucent during the process, due to the slower diffusion rate of ethanol and isopropanol. At higher temperatures (40°C), the shell of microspheres was very thin and some of the microspheres was broken. This effect might be caused by faster diffusion of alcohol in the droplet into aqueous phase and evaporation of dichloromethane immediately after introducing it into the medium.

The polymer concentration in the mixed solvent was another important factor in producing microballoons successfully. It was reported that with increasing the concentration of polymer, the size of the microballoons increased (Kawashima et al., 1991).

The presence of totally hydrolyzed polyvinyl alcohol, employed as an emulsifying agent, significantly prevented aggregation of the droplets with solidified outer shells during the process. It was assumed that the polyvinyl alcohol, adsorbed to the interface between the droplets, and the aqueous medium might form a strong hydrated layer over the droplets, resulting in a stable dispersed system.

The particle size analysis Table (125) showed that the increase in the drug: polymer ratio increased the particle size of the microspheres, that in accordance to the result obtained by Lee et al., 1999 who found that as the amount of Eudragit increased the average particle size together with the wall thickness increased.

The release of metronidazole from floating microspheres at pH 1.2 was shown in Table (122) and Figure (42). It is clear that, the release of the drug was greatly retarded in case of the floating microspheres than that of plain drug. Since the acrylic polymer used is not soluble in acidic pH no significant amount of drug was released from microspheres except for drug: polymer ratio 2:1.

Upon increasing the polymer content in the microspheres from drug: polymer ratio 2:1 to 1:1 to finally 1:2 the release rate decreased from 69.1 to 6.9 and finally to 4.1 % after 6 hours dissolution.

266

Data in Table (123) showed the kinetic treatment of the in-vitro release data of metronidazole from its acrylic floating microspheres. It can be observed that the zero order kinetic controlled the release of metronidazole from its microspheres prepared with Eudragit S in drug: polymer ratios 2:1, 1:1 and 1:2 with t ½ values of 407.75, 3967.447, and 6710.465 min, respectively.

The purpose of preparing floating microspheres is to extend the gastric residence time of the drug. The floating test was carried out to investigate the floatability of the prepared microspheres.

It is clear from Table (124) that most of the prepared microspheres with different drug: polymer ratios were still floated after 6 hours (ranged from 85 to 92 %).This finding indicates that the enteric property of the microballoons shell might be advantageous in prolonging the residence time of microballoons in the stomach. During the floating test, no swelling or gelation of the microballoons was found, which suggested that they could be dispersed individually in the stomach without adhesion to the mucosa.

Conclusion

From the previous results and discussion the following could be concluded:

1-The prepared floating metronidazole capsules complied with the pharmacopeal requirement for uniformity of drug content.

2-The production yield of the prepared metronidazole microspheres was ranged between 43%-59.6%. The loading efficiency percentage was unsatisfactory as it lied between 22.1- 29.5.

3-From the electron microscopic scanning, it was found that the majority of metronidazole microspheres had spherical, regular shape, also showed internal hollow structure which responsible for the floating properties of all the prepared formulae of microspheres for more than 6 hours.

4-Increasing the polymer content in the microspheres from drug: polymer ratio of 2:1 to 1:1 and finally to 1:2 decreased the release rate of drug from 69.1% to 6.9% to 4.1%, respectively.

5-Concerning the buoyancy duration of metronidazole capsule formulae prepared with different eight polymers in different four drug: polymer ratios, only formulae 1cC (capsules containing HPMC 15000 in drug: polymer ratio 2:3), formula 1cD (capsules containing HPMC 15000 in drug: polymer ratio 1:2), formula 2cD(capsules containing HPMC 4000 in drug: polymer ratio 1:2), and formula 8cD (capsules containing pectin in drug: polymer ratio

1:2) that gave promising floating properties as they able to float for 6 hours. While all other formulae showed floating time ranged between 17- 258 minutes.

6-Regarding dissolution study of metronidazole capsule formulae containing HPMC 15000 in four drug: polymer ratios, after 6 hours dissolution, the formula 1cB (containing drug: polymer ratio 1:1) release 94.2% of its drug content, while formula 1cC (containing drug: polymer ratio 2:3) release 93.7% of its drug content and finally formula 1cD (containing drug: polymer ratio 1:2) release 86.6% of its drug content.

7-Concerning dissolution study of metronidazole capsule formulae containing HPMC 4000 in four drug: polymer ratios, after 6 hours dissolution, the formula 2cC (containing drug: polymer ratio 2:3) release 96.5% of its drug content, while formula 2cD (containing drug: polymer ratio 1:2) release 79.5% of its drug content.

8-Regarding dissolution study of metronidazole capsule formulae containing sodium alginate in four drug: polymer ratios, after 6 hours dissolution, only the formula 4cB (containing drug: polymer ratio 1:1) release 87.2% of its drug content.

9-Regarding dissolution study of metronidazole capsule formulae containing CMC in four drug: polymer ratios, after 6 hours dissolution, the formula 5cA (containing drug: polymer ratio 2:1) release 97.4% of its drug content, while formula 5cB (containing drug: polymer ratio 1:1) release 95 % of its drug content, while formula 5cC (containing drug: polymer ratio 2:3) release

269

94.4% of its drug content, and finally formula 5cD (containing drug: polymer ratio 1:2) release 93.1% of its drug content.

10-Regarding dissolution study of metronidazole capsule formulae containing pectin in four drug: polymer ratios, after 6 hours dissolution, both formulae 8cC (containing drug: polymer ratio 2:3) and 8cD (containing drug: polymer ratio 1:2) release all their drug content.

11-While metronidazole capsule formulae prepared with Carbopol 934 showed rapid release of their drug content. Since the maximum retardation effect showed with formulae 3cC (containing drug: polymer ratio 2:3) and formula 3cD (containing drug: polymer ratio 1:2) as they release all their drug content after 2.5 hours.

12-Also, the metronidazole capsule formulae prepared with ethyl cellulose show no significant retardation effect of drug release. The formula 6cD (containing drug: polymer ratio 1:2) release all its drug content after 3 hours.

13-In addition, the metronidazole capsule formulae prepared with methyl cellulose show no significant retardation effect of drug release. Both formula 7cC (containing drug: polymer ratio 2:3) and formula 7cD (containing drug: polymer ratio 1:2) release all their drug content after 3 hours.

14-The following table summarize the best formulae of metronidazole capsule prepared with different ratios of various polymers that gave suitable release after 6 hours and showing their floating duration.

Formulae	Polymer	Drug:polymer ratio	%drug released after 6 hours	Floating duration (hours)
1cB	HPMC 15000	1:1	94.2	2.5
1cC	HPMC 15000	2:3	93.7	6
1cD	HPMC 15000	1:2	86.6	6
2cC	HPMC 4000	2:3	96.5	4.3
2cD	HPMC 4000	1:2	79.5	6
4cB	Sodium alginate	1:1	87.2	0.3
5cA	CMC	2:1	97.4	0.3
5cB	CMC	1:1	95	0.3
5cC	CMC	2:3	94.4	0.3
5cD	CMC	1:2	93.1	0.3
8cC	Pectin	2:3	100	0.3
8cD	pectin	1:2	100	6

15-From the thirty two prepared metronidazole capsule formulae only the following formulae show best results, not only for their drug release but also for being floated for 6 hours, formula 1cC (containing HPMC 15000 in drug: polymer ratio 2:3), formula 1cD (containing HPMC 15000 in drug: polymer ratio 1:2), (formula 2cD (containing HPMC 4000 in drug: polymer ratio 1:2), and finally formula 8cD (containing pectin in drug: polymer ratio 1:2).

16-The in-vitro release of metronidazole from the investigated capsules followed different kinetic orders and no one kinetic order can express the drug release.

17- The in-vitro release of metronidazole from the investigated microspheres followed zero order kinetics.

PART II

Accelerated STABILITY of Metronidazole Floating Dosage Forms

Introduction

The release of a drug from the dosage form into the gastro intestinal fluids is an essential first step in drug absorption and bioavailability (Murthy and Sellerssie, 1993). During storage, a drug product may undergo changes in physicochemical characteristic that can affect the bioavailability of the dosage form which include appearance, chemical assay, degradation product level, moisture content, disintegration time, and dissolution rates (Fung, 1996).

Stability of a pharmaceutical product may be defined as the capability of a particular formulation, in specific container, closure system, to remain within its physical, chemical, microbiological, therapeutic and toxicological specifications (Remington's Pharmaceutical Science, 2000).

Stability of a drug also can be defined as the time from the date of manufacture and packaging of the formulation, until its chemical or biological activity is not less than a predetermined level of a labeled potency, and its physical characteristics have not changed (Remington's Pharmaceutical Science, 2000).

It is true to say that no pharmaceutical product is stable indefinitely and certainly, the majority of products are stable only for a limited time (Pharmaceutical practice, 1990).

An expiration date is then defined as the time in which the preparation will remain stable when stored under recommended conditions (Remington's Pharmaceutical Science, 2000).

The instability of pharmaceutical products may be demonstrated as drug or excipient degradation. All instability is thermodynamic in nature, but poor formulation, poor packaging and poor storage conditions may exacerbate this inherent instability (Pharmaceutical practice, 1990).

Rhodes (1984) has reported six possible results of pharmaceutical product instability. This list is not meant to be fully comprehensive or exhaustive.

1-Loss of active drug.

2-Loss of vehicle.

3-Loss of content uniformity.

4-Reduction in bioavailability (e.g. aging of tablets resulting in a change in dissolution profile).

5-Loss of pharmaceutical elegance (e.g. fading of colored solutions and tablets).

6-Production of potentially toxic materials (e.g. break down products from drug degradation).

It is usual to classify the degradation of pharmaceutical products as being due to chemical, physical and biological mechanisms. In some cases, the degradation may due to one or more of these mechanisms (Pharmaceutical practice, 1990).

Stability study requirements and expiration dating are covered in the Good Manufacturing Practices (cGMPs, 1980), the USP and FDA guidelines (1987). Stable tablets retain their original size, shape, weight, and color under normal handling and storage conditions throughout their shelf life. In addition, the in-vitro availability of the active ingredients should not change appreciably with time (Remington's Pharmaceutical Science, 2000).

Early incompatibilities were quite obvious from the odor of the tablets. Quantitization was another matter, since in the first half of this century quantitative assays to detect such problems relied on some color reaction and colorimeter for quantitation. Spectrophotometers, for all practical purposes, were not easily accessible until the late 1940s.

The introduction of the spectrophotometer on the commercial scale was giant step forward, yet, since many chronophers are common in both parent and decomposition product, specificity was still lacking (Remington's Pharmaceutical Science, 2000).

In 1950s and 1960s, such specificity was supplied in a semi-quantities manner by (TLC). Instead, high precision Liquid Chromatography (HPLC) proved to be the sensor of small amounts of impurity and decomposition product (Jens; Rhodes, 2000).

According to the regulatory definition (cGMPs, 1987), a stability–indicating method is one of a number of quantitative analytical methods that are based on the characteristic structural, chemical, or biological properties of each active ingredient of a drug product and that will distinguish each active ingredient from its degradation products so that the active ingredient content can be accurately measured (Jens and Rhodes, 2000).

276

Non-chromatographic and spectroscopic techniques such as titemetry, atomic adsorption, UV spectrophotometry and infrared spectroscopy, while precise, are not considered stability-indicating, and as such not suitable for stability assessment applications (Jens and Rhodes, 2000).

On the other hand, chromatographic separation methods, such as chiral chromatography (CC), thin-layer chromatography (TLC), and gas chromatography (GC), are stability-indicating and stability-specific methods. Still the most prevalent technique is reversed-phase HPLC alone or with ion-suppression method (Jens and Rhodes, 2000).

The classical method usually employed to determined the stability of new product, is to express the product to ordinary storage conditions(room temperature for the period of time that the product would generally be stored in normal market), e.g., anywhere from two to five years for most pharmaceuticals (Lashman and Cooper, 1959).

The shelf life of many products depends on both the length of time and the temperature during the storage period. The rate of determination of a product on storage is a function of length of storage and temperature during storage (Kowlek and Bookwater, 1971).

Most pharmaceutical decomposition may be due to hydrolysis or oxidation (Martin et al., 1993), this is because most drugs contain more than one functional group, and these may be subjected simultaneously to hydrolysis and oxidation. Other reactions (Mollica, 1978) such as isomerization, epimerization and photolysis may also affect the stability of drugs in the liquid, solid and semisolid products.

1-Hydrolysis

Hydrolysis is considered to be the major cause of deterioration of drug. It may be defined as the reaction of a compound with water, such as the reaction of water with esters as ethyl acetate, and amides as procaine amide. Molecular hydrolysis reactions proceed much slower than the ionic type (protolysis) and its irreversible process results in cleavage of the drug molecule.

The hydrolysis of aspirin was found by Edwards (1950), to be first order and to be catalyzed by hydrogen ions. According to Higuchi et al (1950), procaine decomposes mainly by hydrolysis, the degradation being due to primarily the break down of the unchanged and singly charged forms. The reaction is catalyses by hydroxyl ions. Zuirbis et al (1956) studied the alkaline and acid hydrolysis of atropine and found that the predominant catalytic reaction involved hydroxyl ions above pH 4.5 and hydrogen ions below pH 3. The pH for maximum stability varied between 4.1 at 10°C and 3.2 at 100°C. Kosky (1969) found that the decomposition of salicylamide proceeded by both acid and base catalyzed amide hydrolysis.

2- Oxidation

Oxidation frequently involves free radicals and accompanying chain reactions. These radicals tend to take electrons from other substances and thus bring about oxidation. When a reaction involves molecular oxygen, it is commonly called autoxidation. In most oxidation reactions, the rate is proportional to the concentration of the oxidizing molecule but may be independent on the concentration of oxygen. The reaction is usually catalyzed by the presences of the trace amounts of heavy metals and organic peroxides. Inhibitors or antioxidants act by providing electrons and easily available hydrogen atoms that are accepted by free radicals, and this process stops the chain reaction. The U.S.P permits the addition of a suitable stabilizer such as octochopherol to petrolatum to inhibit oxidation and rancidification (FDA guide lines, 1987).

General Stability Considerations for Metronidazole.

Both metronidazole and metronidazole HCl are stable in air but may darken upon exposure to light (McEvoy, 1995; Martindall, 1993). Product should be packaged in light –resistant containers, and stored at less than 30 °C.

In aqueous media, metronidazole was reported to undergo hydrolysis due to the presence of prototypically generated hydroxyl radicals (Barns et al., 1986). Light irradiation has more effect on the degradation of metronidazole in solution than irradiation with sonic energy (Kendall et al., 1989).

Metronidazole injection should be stored at controlled room temperature and protected from exposure to light and from freezing (McEvoy, 1995;Physician's Desk Reference, 1993). Refrigeration may result crystal formation, but the crystals redissolve upon warming to room temperature (Cano et al., 1986).

279

Reconstituted metronidazole hydrochloride is stable for 96 hours stored below 30°C exposed to normal room light. After dilution in infusion solutions, it should be stored at room temperature and discarded after 24 hours. Refrigeration may result in precipitation (McEvoy, 1995; Martindalle, 1993).

Reconstituted metronidazole hydrochloride reacts with aluminum due to its low pH developing a discoloring variously described as orange, rust, and reddish-brown. Consequently, the use of plastic hub needles is recommended. After dilution and neutralization, the reaction does not occur as readily but may still occur if exposure to aluminum lasts six hours or longer (McEvoy, 1995; Little et al., 1981; Struthers et al., 1985).

Stability Reports of Compounded Products.

Oral products

Mathew et al., (1993) evaluated the stability of metronidazole 5 and 10 mg/ml in several oral liquid dosage forms. Metronidazole content was assessed using an HPLC assay. The liquids prepared from tablets sustained substantial decomposition. Metronidazole 5 mg/ml prepared from powder sustained no loss after 60 days.

Mathew et al., (1994a) also evaluated the stability of benzoate ester of metronidazole prepared as oral suspensions. The metronidazole content was assessed using a stability-indicating HPLC assay. After 90 days of storage at room temperature, there was no loss of metronidazole in either formulation. Further more, the physical properties and pH did not change.

280

Mathew et al., (1994b) evaluated the use of Ora-Plus and Ora-sweet as vehicles for metronidazole oral liquids. Metronidazole tablets were ground to a fine powder and mixed with Ora-Plus or a 1:1 mix of Ora-Sweet to yield 10 mg/ml concentrations. The products were packaged in amber glass bottles and stored at 25°C.Metronidazole content was assessed using a stability-indicating HPLC assay. All oral liquid products retained potency with no measurable loss after 90 days of storage. This result is in contrast to the substantial loss of drug that occurred when water or syrup was used as the vehicle.

Peng et al (1993) investigate the degradation kinetics of metronidazole under various storage conditions such as pH, total buffer concentration, ionic strength, temperature, light exposure, and co solvent system. The stability of metronidazole in solutions containing propylene glycol or polyethylene glycol 400 was also investigated. The degradation rate of metronidazole was invariant under various total buffer concentrations at each specific pH within the investigated pH range. These results indicate that no general acid/base catalysis imposes by acetate, phosphate, and borate buffer species is responsible for the degradation of metronidazole.The maximum stability of metronidazole was at pH 5.6 under zero total buffer species conditions.

Stewart et al., (2000), investigate stability of cefepime hydrochloride injection and metronidazole in poly vinyl chloride bags at different temperatures. Cefepime hydrochloride injection 2 mg was mixed with metronidazole injection USP and metronidazole hydrochloride. The mixtures were stored in polyvinyl chloride bags up to 168 hours at 4,22,and -24C.They found that mixtures of Cefepime and metronidazole in metronidazole injection USP were stable up to 168 hours and 96-168 hours, respectively, stored in PVC bags at 4C.In general, Cefepime and metronidazole controls were more stable than mixtures.

The hydrolysis kinetics of metronidazole amino acid ester prodrugs were studied in aqueous phosphate buffer (pH 7.4) and 80 % human plasma at 37°C (Mahfouz; Hassan, 2001). In all cases, the hydrolysis followed pseudo-first-order kinetics and resulted in a quantitative reversion to metronidazole as evidenced by HPLC analysis. The prodrugs exhibited adequate chemical stability (half life, $t_{1/2}$, 4-16 h) in aqueous phosphate solution of pH 7.4.While in human plasma they were hydrolyzed within a few minutes to metronidazole.

The use of ionizing radiation for sterilization of pharmaceuticals is now a well-established technology. The stability of metronidazole after irradiation have been studied by Basly et al., 1996.Trapped radicals, detectable by electron spin resonance (ESR), appear relatively stable and could be quantified. The formation of radiolytic products was evidenced by HPLC.

In this part, the accelerated stability at 35°C and 45°C for six months, were carried out on the formulated metronidazole dosage forms that gave the best floating and controlled release properties in the previous part, which are:

Formula 1tA (metronidazole tablet containing HPMC 15000 in drug: polymer ratio 2:1),

Formula 2tC (metronidazole tablet containing HPMC 4000 in drug: polymer ratio 2:3),

Formula 3tA (metronidazole tablet containing Carbopol 934 in drug: polymer ratio 2:1),

Formula 5tB (metronidazole tablet containing CMC in drug: polymer ratio 1:1),

Formula 7tA (metronidazole tablet containing methyl cellulose in drug: polymer ratio 2:1),

Formula 8tD (metronidazole tablet containing pectin in drug: polymer ratio 1:2),

Formula 1cC (metronidazole capsule containing HPMC 15000 in drug: polymer ratio 2:3),

Formula 1cD (metronidazole capsule containing HPMC 15000 in drug: polymer ratio 1:2),

Formula 2cD (metronidazole capsule containing HPMC 4000 in drug: polymer ratio 1:2),

Formula 8cD (metronidazole capsule containing pectin in drug: polymer ratio 1:2).

In addition, the accelerated stability of plain tablet and capsule dosage form, which prepared by the same previous method with the same ingredients but without addition of any polymer was done for comparison reason.

By applying some form of Arrhenius equation and substituting the experimentally established specific rate constants at the two elevated temperatures, the energy of activation (E_a) and the decomposition reaction rate constant at room temperature (K_{20}) can be determined. Also, $t_{1/2}$ and t_{90} for each formula can be estimated.

A special computer program was used to determine the kinetic order and kinetic parameters of stability of the investigated metronidazole dosage forms. Zero-, first-, and second order kinetics were tried to choose the suitable order for stability study.

Experimental

Material:

• Concentrated hydrochloric acid, El-Nasr pharmaceutical chemicals Co., Cairo, Egypt.

Equipment:

• Incubators, Heraeus, UT 5060E, West Germany.Two incubators were used and adjusted to 35±1°C and 45±1°C.

• UV Spectrophotometer, JenwayLTD, UK, Felsted, Dunmow, Essex, CM6 3LB, Model 6105 UV/Vis, England.

Methodology:

Method of assay:

Each sample was weighed, powdered (for tablet dosage form) and levigated with 100 ml diluted hydrochloric acid (1 ml in 100 ml H_2O) in 250 ml volumetric flask. Shake the content for 30 minutes, then complete with diluted hydrochloric acid and filtered. The filtrate was diluted quantitively with diluted hydrochloric acid, to obtain a solution having a concentration of about 0.2 mg of metronidazole/ ml. Ten ml of this solution was transferred into 100 ml volumetric flask, diluted to volume with dilute hydrochloric acid, and mixed. The absorbance of this test solution was measured spectrophotometrically at 278 nm using dilute hydrochloric acid as blank. The drug content of the tested sample was determined from the standard calibration curve.

Assessing the validity of the assay method:

This test was made to ensure that the assay is valid method for stability studies, which achieved by the following method:

A known amount of metronidazole was diluted with an equal volume of hydrogen peroxide (20 volume).Also; known amount of metronidazole was diluted with an equal volume of 1.0 M sodium hydroxide solution. The two diluted solutions were left to stand for 48 hours of which a couple of a hours were in direct sunlight. The two solutions were finally assayed for drug content where the decomposition was found to be 100%.

Accelerated stability testing:

Enough samples from each formula were placed in flat dishes, which were left uncovered and stored at temperatures of 35°C and 45°C in thermostatically controlled hot incubators accurate to ±1.0°C. Adequate sample from each formula at each elevated temperature were taken at a time intervals of 0, 14, 30, 45, 60, 90,120 and 180 days. These samples were evaluated according to the method of assay. The method was carried out in triplicate manner for each formula then the mean was taken.

Tables (126-129) showed the results of analysis of undecomposed metronidazole remained in the tested formulae stored at 35°C, and 45°C after different time intervals.

Tables (136-137) demonstrate the metronidazole degradation orders from its tested samples stored at 35°C, and 45°C.

Table (140) reveals the kinetic calculations of the experimental decomposition rate constants K_{35} and K_{45}, as well as, the calculated K_{20} and t $_{90}$ at 20°C.

Figures (47-50) were graphical representations the mean values of the remained metronidazole from its tablets and capsules at 35°C, 45°C experimentally determined during 6 months.

Table (126): Accelerated stability testing of metronidazole tablets stored at 35° C.

formula		Plain tablet	5tB	2tC	1tA	7tA	3tA	8tD
% drug remained after (days)	Zero	100	100	100	100	100	100	100
	7	99.91	99.21	99.81	97.35	99.8	99.34	99.57
	14	99.8	97.71	99.25	97.1	99.25	98.41	97.36
	30	98.1	95	98.88	96.27	98.03	97.15	97.01
	45	97.25	94.37	96.78	95.98	97.15	96.36	95.25
	60	95.01	94.21	96.5	95.11	95.3	96.01	94.98
	90	95.4	90.2	95.53	94.01	93.51	95.21	93.4
	120	94.81	89	94.8	93.3	91.15	94.1	90.21
	180	94	90.9	93.27	92.9	90.34	90.35	88.1

t: tablet dosage form

Plain tablet: (tablet containing the same ingredients without polymer)

5tB: (tablet containing CMC in drug: polymer ratio 1:1)

2tC: (tablet containing HPMC 4000 in drug: polymer ratio 2:3)

1tA: (tablet containing HPMC 15000 in drug: polymer ratio 2:1)

7tA: (tablet containing methyl cellulose in drug: polymer ratio 2:1)

3tA: (tablet containing Carbopol 934 in drug: polymer ratio 2:1)

8tD: (tablet containing pectin in drug: polymer ratio 1:2)

Table (127): Accelerated stability testing of metronidazole tablets stored at 45° C.

formula		Plain tablet	5tB	2tC	1tA	7tA	3tA	8tD
% drug remained after (days)	Zero	100	100	100	100	100	100	100
	7	99.25	99.17	98.71	98.05	99.12	99.01	99.2
	14	97.32	97.35	96.78	98.1	98.33	97.23	97.33
	30	96.91	97.01	95.4	97.23	96.21	95.3	94.3
	45	95.5	95.47	93.21	96.57	95.24	92.31	93.04
	60	94.01	94.71	91.11	94.32	94.8	91.57	91.06
	90	92.7	93.2	90.04	92.2	92.27	90.3	90.1
	120	91.11	91.77	90	90.71	92.11	89.11	88.3
	180	90.21	89.31	88.71	84.1	91.38	88.01	86.71

t: tablet dosage form

Plain tablet: (tablet containing the same ingredients without polymer)

5tB: (tablet containing CMC in drug: polymer ratio 1:1)

2tC: (tablet containing HPMC 4000 in drug: polymer ratio 2:3)

1tA: (tablet containing HPMC 15000 in drug: polymer ratio 2:1)

7tA: (tablet containing methyl cellulose in drug: polymer ratio 2:1)

3tA: (tablet containing Carbopol 934 in drug: polymer ratio 2:1)

8tD: (tablet containing pectin in drug: polymer ratio 1:2)

Table (128): Accelerated stability testing of metronidazole capsules stored at 35° C.

formula		Plain capsule	8cD	1cC	1cD	2cD
% drug remained after (days)	Zero	100	100	100	100	100
	7	99.83	99.81	99.7	99.21	99.65
	14	99.51	99.1	99.23	98.9	99.01
	30	99.01	98.01	98.01	97.37	98.41
	45	98.57	97.23	97.25	96.25	96.91
	60	97.01	96.51	96.41	95.31	95.21
	90	96.11	94.98	95.04	94	93.23
	120	94.25	93.11	93.98	92.21	92.51
	180	93.01	92.01	92.22	90.1	91.11

c: capsule dosage form

Plain capsule: (capsule containing the same ingredients without polymer)

8cD: (capsule containing pectin in drug: polymer ratio 1:2)

1cC: (capsule containing HPMC 15000 in drug: polymer ratio 2:3)

1cD: (capsule containing HPMC 15000 in drug: polymer ratio 1:2)

2cD: (capsule containing HPMC 4000 in drug: polymer ratio 1:2)

Table (129): Accelerated stability testing of metronidazole capsules stored at

45° C.

formula		Plain capsule	8cD	1cC	1cD	2cD
% drug remained after (days)	Zero	100	100	100	100	100
	7	99.7	99.1	99.21	98.9	99.7
	14	98.57	98.03	98	97.37	98.57
	30	97.35	97	97.7	95.81	97.35
	45	96.31	94.27	96.01	94.07	96.31
	60	94.75	92.98	95.3	92.3	94.75
	90	92.87	91.04	94.42	90.15	92.87
	120	91.51	90.1	93.2	89.2	91.51
	180	91.61	80.4	92.51	87.03	91.61

c: capsule dosage form

Plain capsule: (capsule containing the same ingredients without polymer)

8cD: (capsule containing pectin in drug: polymer ratio 1:2)

1cC: (capsule containing HPMC 15000 in drug: polymer ratio 2:3)

1cD: (capsule containing HPMC 15000 in drug: polymer ratio 1:2)

2cD: (capsule containing HPMC 4000 in drug: polymer ratio 1:2)

Table (130): Kinetic parameters for the accelerated stability of metronidazole tablets stored at 35°C and 45°C according to zero-order system.

Formula	35°C					45°C				
	Intercept	Slope	r	k	t½	Intercept	Slope	r	k	t½
Plain tablet	0.851985	0.034623	0.882949	0.034623	1.444.13	1.880075	0.051189	0.951937	0.051189	976.765
5tB	2.660386	0.051496	0.843822	0.051496	970.9458	1.586499	0.053696	0.983147	0.053696	931.1682
2tC	0.576132	0.037676	0.960748	0.037676	1327.114	3.271867	0.054698	0.888788	0.054698	914.1116
1tA	2.861778	0.02763	0.958296	0.02763	1809.651	0.574853	0.080808	0.990732	0.080808	618.7505
7tA	0.392546	0.05923	0.968762	0.05923	844.1655	2.00062	0.044936	0.917842	0.044936	1112.694
3tA	0.960693	0.046492	0.98447	0.046492	1075.461	3.019071	0.060453	0.904677	0.060453	827.0864
8tD	1.213245	0.063506	0.981493	0.063506	787.3326	2.80567	0.068214	0.930706	0.068214	732.9914

t: tablet dosage form

Plain tablet: (tablet containing the same ingredients without polymer)

5tB: (tablet containing CMC in drug: polymer ratio 1:1)   2tC: (tablet containing HPMC 4000 in drug: polymer ratio 2:3)

1tA: (tablet containing HPMC 15000 in drug: polymer ratio 2:1)   7tA: (tablet containing methyl cellulose in drug: polymer ratio 2:1)

3tA: (tablet containing Carbopol 934 in drug: polymer ratio 2:1)   8tD: (tablet containing pectin in drug: polymer ratio 1:2)

Table (131): Kinetic parameters for the accelerated stability of metronidazole tablets stored at 35°C and 45°C according to first-order system.

Formula	35°C					45°C				
	Intercept	Slope	r	k	t ½	Intercept	Slope	r	k	t ½
Plain tablet	1.996301	0.00016	0.88528	0.00036	1937.28	1.991908	0.00024	0.95537	0.00054	1274.8
5tB	1.988304	0.00024	0.84445	0.00055	1262.68	1.993301	0.00025	0.98577	0.00057	1211.71
2tC	1.99758	0.00017	0.96323	0.00039	1773.77	1.985596	0.00026	0.89361	0.00059	1178.67
1tA	1.987438	0.00013	0.9595	0.00029	2381.95	1.998363	0.00038	0.98841	0.00088	784.762
7tA	1.998545	0.00027	0.97067	0.00062	1108.97	1.99129	0.00021	0.92108	0.00047	1461.64
3tA	1.996047	0.00021	0.98456	0.00049	1412	1.986772	0.00028	0.91076	0.00065	1063.72
8tD	1.995063	0.0003	0.98381	0.00068	1018.48	1.987838	0.00032	0.93738	0.00074	936.589

t: tablet dosage form

Plain tablet: (tablet containing the same ingredients without polymer)

5tB: (tablet containing CMC in drug: polymer ratio 1:1)   2tC: (tablet containing HPMC 4000 in drug: polymer ratio 2:3)

1tA: (tablet containing HPMC 15000 in drug: polymer ratio 2:1)   7tA: (tablet containing methyl cellulose in drug: polymer ratio 2:1)

3tA: (tablet containing Carbopol 934 in drug: polymer ratio 2:1)   8tD: (tablet containing pectin in drug: polymer ratio 1:2)

Table (132): Kinetic parameters for the accelerated stability of metronidazole tablets stored at 35°C and 45°C according to second-order system.

Formula	35°C					45°C				
	Intercept	Slope	r	k	t½	Intercept	Slope	r	k	t½
Plain tablet	0.010085	3.7E-06	0.887587	3.7E-06	2705.979	0.010184	5.77E-06	0.958632	5.77E-06	1731.836
5tB	0.010273	5.85E-06	0.844789	5.85E06	1709.067	0.010149	6.09E-06	0.988126	6.09E-06	1641.088
2tC	0.010054	4.05E06	0.965625	4.05E06	2468.396	0.010336	6.32E-06	0.898317	6.32E-06	1581.715
1tA	0.010292	3.06E06	0.960677	3.06E-06	3264.864	0.010015	9.66E-06	0.985515	9.66E-06	1034.731
7tA	0.010027	6.6E-06	0.972248	6.6E-06	1516.28	0.010201	5E-06	0.924216	5E-06	1998.811
3tA	0.010085	5.18E-06	0.984362	5.18E-06	1929.606	0.010307	7.02E-06	0.916681	7.02E-06	1423.549
8tD	0.010105	7.29E-06	0.985785	7.29E-06	1370.893	0.019279	8.03E-06	0.943742	8.03E-06	1244.948

t: tablet dosage form

Plain tablet: (tablet containing the same ingredients without polymer)

5tB: (tablet containing CMC in drug: polymer ratio 1:1)   2tC: (tablet containing HPMC 4000 in drug: polymer ratio 2:3)

1tA: (tablet containing HPMC 15000 in drug: polymer ratio 2:1)   7tA: (tablet containing methyl cellulose in drug: polymer ratio 2:1)

3tA: (tablet containing Carbopol 934 in drug: polymer ratio 2:1)   8tD: (tablet containing pectin in drug: polymer ratio 1:2)

Table (133): Kinetic parameters for the accelerated stability of metronidazole capsules stored at 35°C and 45°C according to zero-order system.

Formula	35°C					45°C				
	Intercept	Slope	r	k	t ½	Intercept	Slope	r	k	t ½
Plain capsule	0.04436	0.042225	0.984691	0.042225	1184.129	1.294796	0.049399	0.925998	0.049399	1012.174
8cD	0.49817	0.046254	0.980605	0.046254	1080.99	0.340566	0.099552	0.981672	0.099552	502.2493
1cC	0.558478	0.043392	0.985232	0.043392	1152.279	1.594689	0.038265	0.946827	0.038265	1306.69
1cD	0.930649	0.053489	0.987521	0.053489	934.7776	2.279738	0.067641	0.958448	0.067641	739.1944
2cD	0.671599	0.052412	0.960343	0.052412	953.9715	0.323281	0.092333	0.989644	0.092333	541.5189

c: capsule dosage form

Plain capsule: (capsule containing the same ingredients without polymer)

8cD: (capsule containing pectin in drug: polymer ratio 1:2)

1cC: (capsule containing HPMC 15000 in drug: polymer ratio 2:3)

1cD: (capsule containing HPMC 15000 in drug: polymer ratio 1:2)

2cD: (capsule containing HPMC 4000 in drug: polymer ratio 1:2)

Table (134): Kinetic parameters for the accelerated stability of metronidazole capsules stored at 35°C and 45°C according to first-order system.

Formula	35°C					45°C				
	Intercept	Slope	r	k	t ½	Intercept	Slope	r	k	t ½
Plain capsule	2.00035	0.00019	0.98556	0.00044	1582.03	1.99444	0.00023	0.92829	0.00052	1333.48
8cD	1.997998	0.00021	0.98223	0.00048	1433.25	1.999986	0.00048	0.97805	0.00111	625.254
1cC	1.997717	0.0002	0.98713	0.00045	1530.54	1.993094	0.00017	0.94954	0.0004	1729.45
1cD	1.996182	0.00025	0.98961	0.00057	1225.14	1.990266	0.00032	0.96309	0.00073	947.287
2cD	1.997248	0.00024	0.96282	0.00055	1258.45	1.999715	0.00044	0.9868	0.00102	680.618

c: capsule dosage form

Plain capsule: (capsule containing the same ingredients without polymer)

8cD: (capsule containing pectin in drug: polymer ratio 1:2)

1cC: (capsule containing HPMC 15000 in drug: polymer ratio 2:3)

1cD: (capsule containing HPMC 15000 in drug: polymer ratio 1:2)

2cD: (capsule containing HPMC 4000 in drug: polymer ratio 1:2)

Table (135): Kinetic parameters for the accelerated stability of metronidazole capsules stored at 35°C and 45°C according to second-order system.

Formula	35°C					45°C				
	Intercept	Slope	r	k	t ½	Intercept	Slope	r	k	t ½
Plain capsule	0.009988	4.54E-06	0.986362	4.54E-06	2200.601	0.010126	5.47E-06	0.930471	5.47E-06	1828.804
8cD	0.010042	5.05E-06	0.983727	5.05E-06	1978.308	0.009966	1.24E-05	0.973249	1.24E-05	808.0277
1cC	0.010049	4.72E-06	0.988905	4.72E-06	2116.499	0.010158	4.2 E-06	0.95179	4.2 E-06	2383.246
1cD	0.010082	5.98E-06	0.991504	5.98E-06	1671.269	0.010219	7.92E-06	0.967472	7.92E-06	1263.032
2cD	0.010059	5.79E-06	0.96521	5.79E-06	1728.097	0.009976	1.13E-05	0.98304	1.13E-05	888.6498

c: capsule containing same ingredients without polymer

Plain capsule: (capsule containing the same ingredients without polymer)

8cD: (capsule containing pectin in drug: polymer ratio 1:2)

1cC: (capsule containing HPMC 15000 in drug: polymer ratio 2:3)

1cD: (capsule containing HPMC 15000 in drug: polymer ratio 1:2)

2cD: (capsule containing HPMC 4000 in drug: polymer ratio 1:2)

Table (136): The calculated correlation coefficients for the accelerated stability of metronidazole tablets and capsules stored at 35°C according to zero-, first- and second-order system.

Order of reaction / Formula	Correlation coefficient (r)		
	Zero-order	First-order	Second-order
Plain tablet	0.882949	-0.88528	0.887587
5tB	0.843822	-0.84445	0.844789
2tC	0.960748	-0.96323	0.965625
1tA	0.958296	-0.9595	0.960677
7tA	0.968762	-0.97067	0.972448
3tA	0.98447	-0.98456	0.984362
8tD	0.981493	-0.98381	0.985785
Plain capsule	0.984691	-0.98556	0.986362
8cD	0.980605	-0.98223	0.983727
1cC	0.985232	-0.98713	0.988905
1cD	0.987521	-0.98961	0.991504
2cD	0.960343	-0.96282	0.96521
Sum	11.47893	-11.49885	11.51698
average	0.956578	-0.958238	0.959748

c: capsule dosage form   t: tablet dosage form

Plain capsule, tablet: (capsule, tablet containing the same ingredients without polymer)

8cD: (capsule containing pectin ratio in 1:2)   1cC: (capsule containing HPMC 15000 in ratio 2:3)

1cD: (capsule containing HPMC 15000 in ratio 1:2)   2cD: (capsule containing HPMC 4000 in ratio 1:2)

5tB: (tablet containing CMC in ratio 1:1)   2tC: (tablet containing HPMC 4000 in ratio 2:3)

1tA: (tablet containing HPMC 15000 in ratio 2:1)   7tA: (tablet containing methyl cellulose in ratio 2:1)

3tA: (tablet containing Carbopol 934 in ratio 2:1)   8tD: (tablet containing pectin in ratio 1:2)

Table (137): The calculated correlation coefficients for the accelerated stability of metronidazole tablets and capsules stored at 45°C according to zero-, first- and second-order system.

Order of reaction / Formula	Correlation coefficient (r)		
	Zero-order	First-order	Second-order
Plain tablet	0.951937	-0.95537	0.958632
5tB	0.983147	-0.98577	0.988126
2tC	0.888788	-0.89361	0.898317
1tA	0.990732	-0.98841	0.985515
7tA	0.917842	-0.92108	0.924216
3tA	0.904677	-0.91076	0.916681
8tD	0.930706	-0.93738	0.943742
Plain capsule	0.925998	-0.92829	0.930471
8cD	0.981672	-0.97805	0.973249
1cC	0.946827	-0.94954	0.952179
1cD	0.985448	-0.96309	0.967472
2cD	0.989644	-0.98680	0.98304
Sum	11.37042	-11.39815	11.42164
average	0.947535	-0.949846	0.951803

c: capsule dosage form   t: tablet dosage form

Plain capsule, tablet: (capsule, tablet containing the same ingredients without polymer)

8cD: (capsule containing pectin ratio in 1:2)   1cC: (capsule containing HPMC 15000 in ratio 2:3)

1cD: (capsule containing HPMC 15000 in ratio 1:2)   2cD: (capsule containing HPMC 4000 in ratio 1:2)

5tB: (tablet containing CMC in ratio 1:1)   2tC: (tablet containing HPMC 4000 in ratio 2:3)

1tA: (tablet containing HPMC 15000 in ratio 2:1)   7tA: (tablet containing methyl cellulose in ratio 2:1)

3tA: (tablet containing Carbopol 934 in ratio 2:1)   8tD: (tablet containing pectin in ratio 1:2)

Table (138): Kinetic parameters for metronidazole tablets and capsules based on accelerated stability testing stored at 35°C according to the suitable kinetic order (second order).

Formula	Intercept	slope	r	K (year)$^{-1}$	t ½ (day)
Plain tablet	0.010085	3.7E-06	0.887587	3.7 E-06	2705.979
5tB	0.010273	5.85 E-06	0.844789	5.85 E-06	1709.067
2tC	0.010054	4.05 E-06	0.965625	4.05 E-06	2468.396
1tA	0.010292	3.06 E-06	0.960677	3.06 E-06	3264.864
7tA	0.010027	6.6 E-06	0.972448	6.6 E-06	1516.28
3tA	0.010085	5.18 E-06	0.984362	5.18 E-06	1929.606
8tD	0.010105	7.29 E-06	0.985785	7.29 E-06	1370.893
Plain capsule	0.009988	4.54 E-06	0.986362	4.54 E-06	2200.601
8cD	0.010042	5.05 E-06	0.983727	5.05 E-06	1978.308
1cC	0.010049	4.72 E-06	0.988905	4.72 E-06	2116.499
1cD	0.010082	5.98 E-06	0.991504	5.98 E-06	1671.269
2cD	0.010059	5.79 E-06	0.96521	5.79 E-06	1728.097

c: capsule dosage form   t: tablet dosage form

Plain capsule, tablet: (capsule, tablet containing the same ingredients without polymer)

8cD: (capsule containing pectin ratio in 1:2)   1cC: (capsule containing HPMC 15000 in ratio 2:3)

1cD: (capsule containing HPMC 15000 in ratio 1:2)   2cD: (capsule containing HPMC 4000 in ratio 1:2)

5tB: (tablet containing CMC in ratio 1:1)   2tC: (tablet containing HPMC 4000 in ratio 2:3)

1tA: (tablet containing HPMC 15000 in ratio 2:1)   7tA: (tablet containing methyl cellulose in ratio 2:1)

3tA: (tablet containing Carbopol 934 in ratio 2:1)   8tD: (tablet containing pectin in ratio 1:2)

Table (139): Kinetic parameters for metronidazole tablets and capsules based on accelerated stability testing stored at 45°C according to the suitable kinetic order (second order).

Formula	Intercept	slope	r	K (year)$^{-1}$	t ½ (day)
Plain tablet	0.01010184	5.77E-06	0.958632	5.77 E-06	1731.836
5tB	0.010149	6.09E-06	0.988126	6.09E-06	1641.088
2tC	0.010336	6.32 E-06	0.898317	6.32E-06	1581.715
1tA	0.010015	9.66 E-06	0.985515	9.66E-06	1034.731
7tA	0.010201	5E-06	0.924216	5E-06	1998.811
3tA	0.010307	7.02 E-06	0.916681	7.02E-06	1423.549
8tD	0.010279	8.03 E-06	0.943742	8.03E-06	1244.948
Plain capsule	0.010126	5.47 E-06	0.930471	5.47E-06	1828.804
8cD	0.009966	1.24E-05	0.973249	1.24E-05	808.0277
1cC	0.010158	4.2E-06	0.952179	4.2E-06	2383.246
1cD	0.010219	7.92E-06	0.967472	7.92E-06	1263.032
2cD	0.009976	1.13E-05	0.98304	1.13E-05	888.6498

c: capsule dosage form   t: tablet dosage form

Plain capsule, tablet: (capsule, tablet containing the same ingredients without polymer)

8cD: (capsule containing pectin ratio in 1:2)   1cC: (capsule containing HPMC 15000 in ratio 2:3)

1cD: (capsule containing HPMC 15000 in ratio 1:2)   2cD: (capsule containing HPMC 4000 in ratio 1:2)

5tB: (tablet containing CMC in ratio 1:1)   2tC: (tablet containing HPMC 4000 in ratio 2:3)

1tA: (tablet containing HPMC 15000 in ratio 2:1)   7tA: (tablet containing methyl cellulose in ratio 2:1)

3tA: (tablet containing Carbopol 934 in ratio 2:1)   8tD: (tablet containing pectin in ratio 1:2)

Table (140): Kinetic data for metronidazole tablets and capsules based on accelerated stability testing.

Formula	K_{35} (days)$^{-1}$	K_{45} (days)$^{-1}$	k_{20} (days)$^{-1}$	Ea cal/mole	$t_{½}$ at 20°C(day)	t_{90} at 20°C(day)
Plain tablet	3.7E-06	5.77 E-06	1.79491	8649.055	5571.312	618.4156
5tB	5.85E-06	6.09 E-06	5.4793	782.6172	1825.035	202.5788
2tC	4.05 E-06	6.32 E-06	1.96258	8661.961	5095.338	565.5825
1tA	3.06 E-06	9.66 E-06	4.70192	22376.53	21235.38	2357.127
7tA	6.6 E-06	5 E-06	1.03174	5404.1	964.1916	107.0253
3tA	5.18 E-06	7.02 E-06	3.15808	5916.539	3166.478	351.479
8tD	7.29 E-06	8.03 E-06	6.22833	1881.893	1605.567	178.2179
Plain capsule	4.54 E-06	5.47 E-06	3.35197	3627.33	2983.318	331.1482
8cD	5.05 E-06	1.24 E-05	1.16994	17485.55	8547.428	948.7645
1cC	4.72 E-06	4.2 E-06	5.7078	2272.04	1751.987	194.4706
1cD	5.98 E-06	7.92 E-06	3.78484	5469.088	2642.118	293.2751
2cD	5.79 E-06	1.13 E-05	1.94945	13015.66	5129.659	569.3921

c: capsule dosage form   t: tablet dosage form

Plain capsule, tablet: (capsule, tablet containing the same ingredients without polymer)

8cD: (capsule containing pectin ratio in 1:2)   1cC: (capsule containing HPMC 15000 in ratio 2:3)

1cD: (capsule containing HPMC 15000 in ratio 1:2)   2cD: (capsule containing HPMC 4000 in ratio 1:2)

5tB: (tablet containing CMC in ratio 1:1)   2tC: (tablet containing HPMC 4000 in ratio 2:3)

1tA: (tablet containing HPMC 15000 in ratio 2:1)   7tA: (tablet containing methyl cellulose in ratio 2:1)

3tA: (tablet containing Carbopol 934 in ratio 2:1)   8tD: (tablet containing pectin in ratio 1:2)

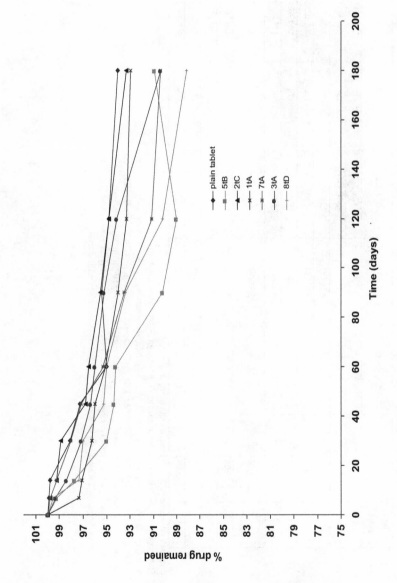

Figure (47): Percent remained of metronidazole from its tablet formulae stored at 35°C.

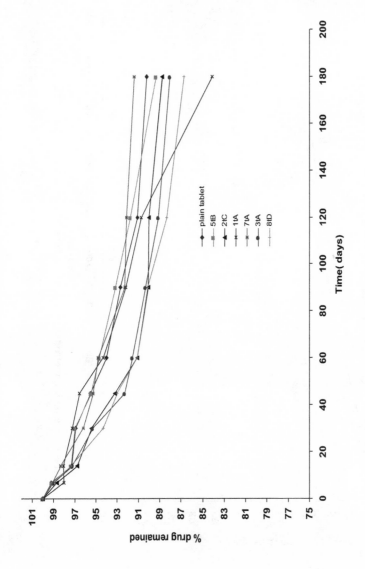

Figure (48): Percent remained of metronidazole from its tablet formulae stored at 45°C .

304

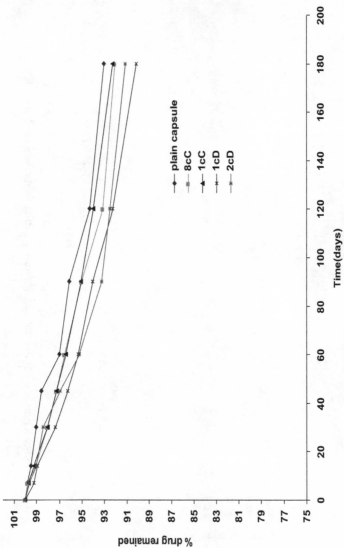

Figure (49): Percent remained of metronidazole from its capsule formulae stored at 35°C.

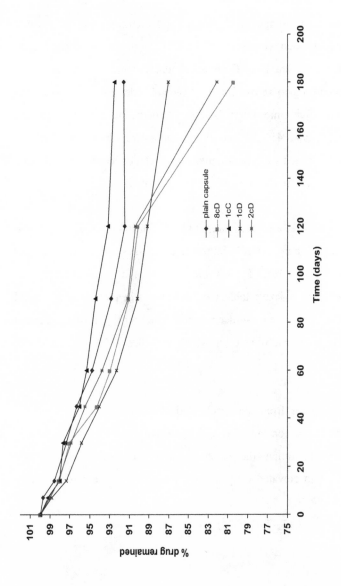

Figure (50): Percent remained of metronidazole from its capsule formulae stored at 45°C.

306

Results and Discussion

The effect of storage of the formulated metronidazole tablets and capsules at two elevated temperatures 35°, 45°C on the chemical stability of metronidazole was studied. Correlation coefficient (r) values were determined according to zero-, first- and second order equations using the remained drug after time intervals for 6 months at the two elevated temperatures (35 and 45 °C) and the decomposition rate constant was determined according to the most suitable correlation coefficient. Kinetic treatments and kinetic parameters were also calculated.

Tables (126-129) and Figures (47-50) illustrated the accelerated stability testing of metronidazole tablets and capsules at the two elevated temperatures 35°C and 45°C. From Tables (136-137), it was obvious that the degradation of metronidazole tablets and capsules when stored at 35°C and 45°C was found to be second-order reaction based on the most appropriate value of correlation coefficient (r) which was 0.959748 and 0.951803, respectively.

It was possible from the accelerated stability data to calculate the specific reaction rate constants k_{35} and k_{45} using some form of Arrhenius equation and substituting the experimentally established specific rate constant at the two elevated temperatures, the energy of activation can be determined as follow:

Log k_2/k_1=Ea/2.303R $(T_2-T_1)/ (T_2T_1)$

Where:

K_1: specific reaction rate constant at temperature t_1.

K_2: specific reaction rate constant at temperature t_2.

Ea: energy of activation.

R: gas constant (1.9872 cal/mole).

T_1: absolute temperature for t_1 (t_1+273).

T_2: absolute temperature for t_2 (t_2+273).

In this way, it will be possible to predict decomposition reaction rate constant at room temperature (Garret, 1956), k_{20}, by a second substitution in the Arrhenius equation using the determined activation energy and one of the elevated temperature rate constant. By knowing k_{20}, it was possible calculate the half –life, ($t_{1/2}$), as well as, the time after which the tablets lost 10 % of their initial contents. The later value t $_{90}$, is a direct interpretation of the length of time through which the tablets would remained complying official requirements of drug contents.

Table (126) and Figure (47) showed the results of accelerated stability testing of metronidazole tablets stored at 35°C within 180 days. The percent of drug remained after 180 days were 90.9, 93.27, 92.9, 90.34, 90.35, 88.1and 94 for formula 5tB, 2tC, 1tA, 7tA, 3tA, 8tD and plain tablets, respectively.

Table (127) and Figure (48) showed the results of accelerated stability testing of metronidazole tablets stored at 45°C within 180 days. The percent of drug remained after 180 days were 89.31, 88.71, 84.1, 91.38, 88.01, 86.71

and 90.21% for formula 5tB, 2tC, 1tA, 7tA, 3tA, 8tD and plain tablets, respectively.

Tables (130-132) illustrated the kinetic parameters of metronidazole tablet formulae (intercept, slope, r, k, and t ½) at zero-, first- and second-order system.

Table (128) and Figure (49) showed the results of accelerated stability testing of metronidazole capsules stored at 35°C within 180 days. The percent of drug remained after 180 days were 92.01, 90.1, 92.22, 91.11 and 93.01 for formula 8cD, 1cC, 1cD, 2cD and plain capsules, respectively.

Table (129) and Figure (50) showed the results of accelerated stability testing of metronidazole capsules stored at 45°C within 180 days. The percent of drug remained after 180 days were 80.4, 87.03, 92.51, 82.1 and 91.61 for formula 8cD, 1cC, 1cD, 2cD and plain capsules, respectively.

Tables (133-135) illustrated the kinetic parameters of metronidazole capsule formulae (intercept, slope, r, k, and t ½) at zero-, first- and second-order system.

So, the degradation of metronidazole tablets and capsules studied were arranged, in descending manner , according to the accelerated stability testing, when stored at 35°C for 180 days, as follows: plain metronidazole tablets > formula 2tC (tablet containing HPMC 4000 in drug: polymer ratio 2:3) > plain metronidazole capsules > formula 1tA(tablet containing HPMC 15000 in drug: polymer ratio 2:1) > formula 1cC(capsule containing HPMC

309

15000 in drug: polymer ratio 2:3) > formula 8cD (capsule containing pectin in drug: polymer ratio 1:2) > formula 2cD(capsule containing HPMC 4000 in drug: polymer ratio 1:2) > formula 5tB (tablet containing CMC in drug: polymer ratio 1:1) > formula 3tA(tablet containing Carbopol 934 in drug: polymer ratio 2:1) > formula 7tA(tablet containing methyl cellulose in drug: polymer ratio 2:1) > formula 1cD(capsule containing HPMC 15000 in drug: polymer ratio 1:2) > formula 8tD(tablet containing pectin in drug: polymer ratio 1:2).

While the degradation of metronidazole tablets and capsules studied were arranged, in descending manner, according to the accelerated stability testing, after being stored at 45°C for 180 days, as follows: formula 1cC (capsule containing HPMC 15000 in drug: polymer ratio 2:3) > plain metronidazole capsule > formula 7tA (tablet containing methyl cellulose in drug: polymer ratio 2:1) > plain metronidazole tablet > formula 5tB(tablet containing CMC in drug: polymer ratio 1:1) > formula 2tC (tablet containing HPMC 4000 in drug: polymer ratio 2:3) > formula 3tA(tablet containing Carbopol 934 in drug: polymer ratio 2:1) > formula 1cD (capsule containing HPMC 15000 in drug: polymer ratio 1:2) > formula 8tD(tablet containing pectin in drug: polymer ratio 1:2) > formula 1tA(tablet containing HPMC 15000 in drug: polymer ratio 2:1) > formula 2cD(capsule containing HPMC 4000 in drug: polymer ratio 1:2) > formula 8cD(capsule containing pectin in drug: polymer ratio 1:2).

Table (136) shows the correlation coefficient (r) values based on kinetic treatment for the accelerated stability testing of metronidazole tablets and capsules stored at 35°C according to zero-, first- and second-order

310

systems. While Table (137) illustrated the correlation coefficient (r) values based on kinetic treatment for the accelerated stability testing of metronidazole tablets and capsules stored at 45°C according to zero-, first- and second-order systems. Tables (138-139) showed the kinetic parameters for metronidazole tablets and capsules based on accelerated stability testing at 35°C and 45°C according to the suitable kinetic order (second order).

Table (140) illustrates the kinetic data for metronidazole tablets and capsules based on accelerated stability testing. The table contains the values of Ea, calculated k_{20}, the values of t $_{90}$ and t ½ at 20°C for all tested formulae.

Metronidazole tablets and capsules studied were arranged, in descending manner, according to t $_{90}$ at 20°C, as follows: formula 1tA(tablet containing HPMC 15000 in drug: polymer ratio 2:1) > formula 8cD(capsule containing pectin in drug: polymer ratio 1:2) > plain metronidazole tablet > formula 2cD(capsule containing HPMC 4000 in drug: polymer ratio 1:2) > formula 2tC (tablet containing HPMC 4000 in drug: polymer ratio 2:3) > formula 3tA(tablet containing Carbopol 934 in drug: polymer ratio 2:1) > plain metronidazole capsule> formula 1cD(capsule containing HPMC 15000 in drug: polymer ratio 1:2) > formula 5tB(tablet containing CMC in drug: polymer ratio 1:1) > formula 1cC(capsule containing HPMC 15000 in drug: polymer ratio 2:3) > formula 8tD(tablet containing pectin in drug: polymer ratio 1:2) > formula 7tA(tablet containing methyl cellulose in drug: polymer ratio 2:1) .

311

Generally, the long t $_{90}$ indicates high stability of metronidazole in the investigated formulae. This high stability may explain that no interference or complexation occurs between metronidazole and other excepients in the same formula. However, the shortest t $_{90}$ indicate higher rate of decomposition.

Conclusion

On evaluating the whole set of results obtained in the present accelerated stability testing, one can observe the formula 1tA (tablet containing HPMC 15000 in drug: polymer ratio 2:1) had the longest t $_{90}$ among all the other formulae studied, while formula 7tA (tablet containing methyl cellulose in drug: polymer ratio 2:1) had the shortest t $_{90}$.

PART III

Bioavailability

Of Metronidazole floating

dosage forms

Introduction

Bioavailability and bioequivalence are two of the important issues taken into consideration in the development of any new products. For systemically delivered oral products, bioavailability is a measure of the rate and extent (total amount) of drug absorption into the general circulation from an administered dosage form. Bioequivalence, on the other hand, means that the drug absorption from a test dosage form is comparable in the rate and the extent as from a reference standard product. To establish bioequivalence, it often requires the measurement of drug and/ or metabolite level either in the blood or in urine over a fixed time period following the administration of different drug dosage forms (Su et al., 1991).

The bioavailability is a term used to indicate the rate and the relative amount of the administered drug which reach the general circulation intact.Therefore bioavailability must include not only how much of the active ingredient is available during dosage, but also the manner at which it is available (Notari, 1971).

Relative bioavailability is the bioavailability of a given drug from a 'test' dosage form compared to the bioavailability of the same drug administered in a 'standard' dosage form which is either an orally administered solution of the drug (from which the drug is known to be well absorbed) or an established commercial preparation of proven clinical effectiveness. Hence relative bioavailability is a measure of the fraction (or percentage) of a given drug that is absorbed intact into the systemic circulation from a dosage form relative to recognized (i.e., clinically proven) standard dosage form of that drug. The relative bioavailability of a given drug administered as equal doses of a test dosage form and a recognized standard dosage form, respectively, by the same route of administration to the same subject on different occasions may be calculated from the corresponding plasma concentration-time curves as follows:

Relative bioavailability = $(AUC_T)_{test}$/dose ÷ $(AUC_T)_{standard}$/dose

Where $(AUC_T)_{test}$ and $(AUC_T)_{standard}$ are the total areas under the plasma concentration-time curves following administration of a single dose of the test dosage form and the standard dosage form, respectively (Michael, 1990).

There are several direct and indirect methods of assessing bioavailability. The selection of a method depends upon the purpose of the study, the analytical method of drug measurement and the nature of the drug product. Blood level, urine excretion data, acute pharmacological response and clinical observation are utilized for assessment of bioavailability (Shargel and Yu, 1999).

By understanding the in-vivo release kinetics of a drug in the gastro intestinal tract, delivery of the drug from the dosage form can be designed accordingly. The purpose of our study was, therefore, to determine the in-vivo performance of the selected floating dosage forms with controlled release of metronidazole. The investigation was a pharmacokinetic evaluation of the selected formulation, which provides an indirect assessment of release and subsequent absorption in the gastro intestinal tract for metronidazole. Therefore, during the subsequent section, pharmacokinetic and detection methods of metronidazole in different biological samples are going to be summarized.

Metronidazole   [1-(2hydroxyethyl)-2-methyl-5-nitroimidazole, Figure (6) is widely used for the treatment of protozoal and anaerobic bacterial infections (Brogden et al., 1978, Ralph, 1983).It is also used in combination therapy with other antibiotics and/or acid-suppressing agents for the treatment of gastric Helicobacter Pylori infections. Metronidazole is also gaining wider use in the treatment of Crohn's disease, a depilating enteritis (Brandt et al., 1982).

In human liver, metronidazole is extensively metabolized primarily by as yet not fully identified cytochrome(s) P 450 (Loft et al., 1991), giving rise to two principal metabolites: the   1-(2-hydroxyethyl)-2-hydroxymethyl-5nitroimidazole (hydroxymetronidazole, figure 1) and 2-methyl-5-nitroimidazole-1-acetic acid (Stambaugh et al., 1986). The acetic acid metabolite only found in urine and dose not posses any pharmacological activity (Haller, 1982; O'keefe et al., 1982). However, hydroxymetronidzole has, against certain strains of bacteria, an antimicrobial potency approximately 30% that of metronidazole (Ralph et al., 1975) and can be detected readily in the systemic circulation.

Glucuronidation and renal excretion of the unchanged compound are minor elimination pathways. Elimination occurs mainly by renal excretion of the metabolites (60-80% of total dose); faecal excretion accounts for only 6 to 15 % of total dose (Rosenblatt and Randall, 1987).

Metronidazole   Hydroxymetronidazole

Figure (50): Chemical structures of metronidazole and hydroxymetronidazole.

A large number of high-performance liquid chromatographic methods have been described to analyze metronidazole in body fluids.

A rapid, selective and sensitive HPLC assay has been developed for the routine analysis of metronidazole in small volumes of rat plasma, gastric aspirate and gastric tissue (Wibawa et al., 2001). The extraction procedure involves liquid-liquid extraction and a protein precipitation step. The measured recovery was at least 78% in all sample matrices. The method proved robust and reliable when applied to the measurement of metronidazole in rat plasma, gastric juice aspirate and gastric tissue for pharmacokinetic studies in individual rats.

Mahfouz and Hassan, 2001, have evaluated bioavailability of metronidazole amino acid ester prodrugs in rabbits. In-vivo experiments in rabbits revealed a higher metronidazole plasma level with sustained release characteristics within the prodrug-treated animals as compared with the parent drug-treated group. In conclusion, the designed amino

317

acid esters 3a and 3c-e might be considered as good candidates for water –soluble prodrug forms of metronidazole.

Rajnarayana et al., 2003, have made before/after non-blinded investigation conducted in healthy male volunteers to screen for inhibitory effects of diosmin on cytochrome p (450) - mediated metabolism of metronidazole. Serum concentrations of metronidazole up to 48 hour post dose, and urinary concentrations of metronidazole and its two major metabolites up to 24 hours post dose were measured using reversed-phase high –performance liquid chromatography. Diosmin pretreatment significantly altered the metabolism of metronidazole, as demonstrated by changes in plasma pharmacokinetics as well as by urinary recovery of both parent drug and its major metabolites. This may be caused by the inhibition of cytochrome p (450) enzyme.

Study on the influence of silymarin pretreatment on metabolism and disposition of metronidazole have been made by Rajnrayana et al., 2004. A clinical study was under taken in 12 healthy volunteers. At first, subjects received metronidazole alone for 3 days. On day 4, blood and urine were collected and metabolism levels were measured. After washout period of one week, silymarin was given for 9 days. On day 10, blood and urine were collected and levels of metronidazole and its metabolite were measured by HPLC. The results revealed that the administration of silymarin increase the clearance of metronidazole and its major metabolite, hydroxy-metronidazole (HM), with a concomitant decrease in half-life, C max and AUC (0-48).

The evaluation of metronidazole and its main metabolite concentrations in the skin after a single oral dose were studied (Bielecka

318

and Klimowicz, 2003).A single oral dose of 2 g of the parent drug was administered to 10 healthy male volunteers. Also microdialysis probes ere inserted intradermally. Drug and metabolite concentrations were measured by HPLC. The results indicate that C_{max}, AUC, and t_{max} in plasma, cutaneous microdialysates and theoretical peripheral compartment did not differ significantly.

The pharmacokinetic evaluation of metronidazole in guar-gum based colon targeted oral drug delivery system was evaluated in healthy volunteers by Krishnaiah et al., 2003.This study was carried out to find the in vivo performance of guar gum-based colon targeted tablets of metronidazole compared to an immediate release tablets in human volunteers. Blood samples were obtained and plasma concentrations of metronidazole were estimated by reverse phase HPLC. The AUC $_{0-\infty}$ and $t_{1/2}$ of metronidazole were unaltered on administrating the drug as a colon-targeted tablet indicating that the extent of absorption and elimination were mot affected by targeting the drug to the colon.

In vitro release and vaginal absorption of metronidazole suppositories in rabbits have been evaluated by Ozyazici et al., 2003.Vaginal suppositories formulations of metronidazole were prepared using six bases as Witepsol H15, Cremao, Ovucire WL 2944, Ovucire WL 3264, PEG 1500 and PEG 6000. The results of this study suggest that the Ovucire WL 3264 suppository of metronidazole prepared for vaginal infection could also be effective in the urinary infections.

Gascon et al., 2003, have evaluated the pharmacokinetic and tissue penetration of metronidazole plus pefloxacin after administration as surgical prophylaxis in colorectal surgery. Metronidazole and pefloxacin were administered as an intravenous infusion 1 hour before surgery. Mean plasma levels, and mean tissue levels of both drug were measured. The results indicate that, the concentration of metronidazole and pefloxacin as prophylactic agents produce plasma and tissue levels above the MIC values of the main pathogens responsible for this kind of infection.

99mTc-labeling studies of a modified metronidazole and its biodistribution in tumor bearing animal models have been investigated by Das et al., 2003. A cysteine-based bifunctional chelating agent with a free carboxylic acid group was synthesized. This chelating agent was coupled to metronidazole. The (99m)Tc labeling studies of the novel agent thus obtained. Biodistribution studies showed selective accumulation of the injected activity in the tumor with renal as well as hepatobiliary clearance. High tumor/muscle ratio of the novel agent indicates considerable promise towards further evaluation.

Metronidazole is synthetic nitroimidazole-derived anti-bacterial and anti-protozoal agent used for the treatment of infection involving gram-negative anaerobes. Tsai and Chen, 2003 have developed an in vivo microdialysis with microbore HPLC system for the pharmacokinetic study of metronidazole in rat blood, brain and bile. In addition, to investigate the disposition mechanism of metronidazole, the p-glycoprotein modulator and cytochrome p (450) inhibitor were concomitantly administered. The findings suggest that metronidazole penetrate the blood-brain barrier (BBB) and goes through hepatobiliary excretion.

Tissue diffusion of metronidazole according to two routes of administration: intravenous and rectal was studied (Jacoberger et al., 2000). Plasma and tissue concentrations were determined by HPLC.The rectal route seems less effective than the IV route, indeed 25%of patients show tissue rate greater or equal to MIC 90%against 89%for the IV route.

A series of identical twin esters 3a-e of metronidazole was synthesized and evaluated as potential prodrugs with improved physicochemical and pharmacokinetic properties (Mahfouz et al., 1998). Reversion kinetics of the parent drug from its twin esters was investigated in aqueous buffer solution as well as in biological media using HPLC.In-vivo evaluation studies of metronidazole and its twin esters 3a-d in mice and 3b in rabbits revealed that the prodrugs have been absorbed almost unhydrolyzed with considerable higher plasma level.

Galmier et al., 1998, have developed a simple and sensitive HPLC method for determination of metronidazole in human plasma. A step of freezing the protein precipitate allowed an efficient separation of aqueous and organic phases minimizing the noise level and improved therefore the limit of quantitation (10 ng/ml using 1 ml of plasma sample). Metronidazole was well resolved from the plasma constituents and internal standard. An excellent linearity was observed between peak-height ratios plasma concentrations over a concentration range of 0.01 to 10 ug/ml. The method is suitable for bioavailability and pharmacokinetic studies in humans.

Antibiotics, which are actively secreted into gastric fluid, may be more efficacious in the eradication of Helicobacter pylori in peptic ulcer disease. Other agents used in the treatment of this disease such as omeprazole may alter the secretion and/or distribution characteristics of

321

antibiotics. In order to test the applicability of these concepts to metronidazole, a sensitive and specific HPLC assay was developed to quantitate omeprazole in plasma, and metronidazole in plasma and gastric fluid (Yeung et al., 1998). Metronidazole, and omeprazole were well separated and recoveries in plasma were greater than 80%. Using 0.3 ml of sample, the assay sensitivity was less than 0.1 µg/ml and linear up to 10 µg/ml. It was applied successfully in determining metronidazole concentrations in clinical samples of plasma and gastric fluid.

David et al., 1998, also have studied the effect of a 5-day administration of omeprazole on metronidazole pharmacokinetics. The study had an open, randomized, two-period crossover design with a 21-day washout period between the phases. Plasma concentrations of metronidazole and its hydroxy-metabolite were measured by reversed phase HPLC with ultraviolet detection. The results indicate that short-term treatment with omeprazole in healthy volunteers does not alter the extent or the rate of metronidazole absorption, and does not affect metronidazole clearance.

Topical metronidazole is effective in the treatment of papulopustular rosacea, a common inflammatory disease of the face. Comparison of the bioavailability of two topical formulations (A and B) of 0.75%metronidazole has been mad by Dykes et al., 1997.The tissue were extracted and analyzed by an HPLC method. Both formulations showed rapid percutaneous penetration. Formulation A clearly gives a higher rate of percutaneous penetration leading to higher tissue levels of drug.

322

A liquid chromatography assay for the study of serum and gastric juice metronidazole concentrations in the treatment of Helicobacter pylori was investigated by Pollak 1996.Using an isocratic HPLC method, with 8 –min run time and protein precipitation of samples, metronidazole could be measured reliably to as low as 0.5 mg/ml in 100 u ml samples of serum, gastric juice, or saliva. The range and accuracy of the assay proved to be suitable for carrying out pharmacokinetic studies at clinically used doses of the drug.

To date, the effect of sucralfate on the pharmacokinetic of nitroimidazole compounds used in triple therapy such as metronidazole is unknown. Amaral-Moraes et al., 1996, have investigated the effect of a 5-day administration period of sucralfate on metronidazole pharmacokinetics. Fourteen healthy male volunteers were selected. The plasma concentration of metronidazole and its hydroxy-metabolite were measured by reversed phase HPLC.The results indicate that no statistically significant difference was observed in any of the pharmacokinetic parameters studied in the absence and presence of sucralfate.

A rapid and selective HPLC method has been developed for the separation and quantitation of metronidazole and its hydroxylated metabolite in human plasma, saliva and gastric juice (Jessa et al., 1996). The assay requires a simple protein precipitation step selective, sensitive and reproducible.

Muscara et al., 1995, investigate the metronidazole pharmacokinetics in patients with different degrees of liver cirrhosis (A, B or C as liver disease severity increases) and in schistosomic patients.

The plasma concentrations of metronidazole and its metabolite were quantified by reversed phase HPLC with UV detection. Comparison of the metronidazole AUC_{0-24} h, $t_{1/2}$ and CL values revealed that metronidazole metabolism is progressively impaired as the severity of liver disease increase. These results indicate that the clinical assessment of liver disease is parallel by an impairment of metronidazole metabolism.

Bioavailability of vagimid 500 tablets (film coated, 500 mg metronidazole) and absorption of metronidazole into the systemic circulation after vaginal administration of vagimid vaginal tablets (100 mg metronidazole) were studied in 16 female healthy volunteers (Hoffmann et al., 1995). Metronidazole and its main hydroxylated metabolite were measured using an HPLC-method with detection limits of 0.025 and 0.25 µg/ml (for vaginal and oral studies) respectively. The absorption of metronidazole into the systemic circulation after vaginal administration of vagimid vaginal tablets caused maximal serum concentrations between433 and 1,156 ng/ml after 8-20 hour which are bactericidal only for the most susceptible anaerobic germs and which are most likely only of marginal importance for the drug safety.

Pargal et al., 1993, have made comparative pharmacokinetics and amoebicidal activity of metronidazole and satranidazole in golden hamster. Blood and liver samples were collected at frequent time intervals and assayed for metronidazole and satranidazole by HPLC.The comparative liver pharmacokinetics parameters C_{max}, t_{max}, and $t_{1/2}$ did not differ significantly.

Siegmund et al., 1992 investigate the bioavailability of metronidazole (0.5g) from vagimidR tablets and compared with tablets of a reference formulation in 12 male healthy volunteers. Metronidazole and its two main oxidized metabolites in serum were determined quantitively with an HPLC method. Metronidazole from vagimidR tablets was absorbed more rapidly than from the reference but at the same extent of absorption.

Metronidazole concentrations in plasma were measured by HPLC in 12 healthy female volunteers after single and repeated vaginal administrations of 500 mg metronidazole pessaries (Salas-Herrera et al., 1991). The plasma concentration of metronidazole at steady state was above the minimum inhibitory concentration (MIC) for anaerobic streptococci and Clostridium tetani. These results demonstrate much lower systemic exposure than after oral administration.

Most of the available pharmacokinetic data were obtained when the drug was administered at the low end of the dosage range. Several other studies were done using assay that were subject to interference by metabolites. Pharmacokinetics of intravenous metronidazole at different dosages in healthy subjects in a crossover manner was evaluated using HPLC assay (Lau et al., 1991). Analysis of variance revealed a statistically significant difference between the low dose (250 mg) and the high dose (1.0 gm and 2.0 gm) effect on the calculated pharmacokinetic parameters. These findings revealed that the pharmacokinetics of metronidazole and its hydroxy metabolites are altered when higher doses of the drug are given; the metabolic transformation of the parent drug is also expected to be reduced.

The influence of prednisolone, sulfasalzine, cimetidine, and Phenobarbital on the pharmacokinetics of metronidazole was investigated in six Crohn's patients (Eradiri et al., 1988). Plasma and urine samples were analyzed for the drug and its two principle metabolites, hydroxymetronidazole and metronidazole-1-acetic acid, by HPLC.This study was reflected insignificant increases in the renal clearance of metronidazole and AUC of the hydroxy metabolite as well as significant decreases in AUC, half-life, and urinary excretion of the parent drug.

Simultaneous determination of metronidazole and chloroquine in human biological fluid has been done using HPLC method with UV detection (Okonkwo et al., 1988). The assay system was found flexible and economical for the therapeutic monitoring of these two important tropical drugs.

The pharmacokinetics and metabolism of intravenous metronidazole were studied in six patients with acute renal failure (Somogyi et al., 1984). Plasma concentrations of metronidazole and its hydroxy and acetic acid metabolites were measured by a specific and sensitive HPLC method. In the patients studied, a dosing regimen of 500 mg twice daily resulted in therapeutically adequate blood levels of metronidazole.

Kaye et al., 1980 developed a rapid and specific HPLC assay for the measurement of metronidazole levels in small volumes of plasma, saliva, serum, urine and whole blood. The method is sufficiently sensitive for monitoring Flagyl therapy in these biological fluids and for pharmacokinetic studies with Flagyl up to at least 24 hours after a single

400 mg oral dose. Furthermore, the method is also capable of assaying two major oxidative metabolites of metronidazole.

The aim of the following work is to study the bioavailability of the prepared selected metronidazole capsules and tablets as compared to commercially available product namely flagyl tablets(El amrya.Co) after their oral administration to human volunteers.

The pharmacokinetic parameters of different metronidazole treatments administrated orally to human volunteers have been calculated. Also the relative bioavailability of the prepared dosage forms compared to the commercial product was estimated.

EXPERIMENTAL

Material:

- Metronidazole, acetonitrile, $ZnSO_4$, ethanol, and potassium dihydrogen phosphate (HPLC grade) were kindly supplied by 10th of Ramadan Company.
- Tinidazole was kindly supplied by MUP pharmaceutical company. N.B All the used materials were of analytical grade.
- Commercially available metronidazole, Flagyl tablet batch no. 2502085, Alexandria Pharmaceutical Co.Alexandria, Egypt.

Equipment:

- The chromatography was carried out using an HP1100 instrument (Hewlett-Packard,les Ulis,UK) equipped with power supplier, an auto sampler and UV spectrophotometric detector connecting to data collection system. The analytical column used was LIChrospher 100RP18 (Sum Putielesize, 125x4 mm) from Merch.
- Vortex mixer, Medtronic, P-selecta, 246539, Switzerland.
- Centrifuge Janetzki T30, Germany.
- Deep freezer, General electric, 500 P123, USA.

328

Methodology:

1-Treatments:

Treatment (1): using commercial tablet containing 250 mg metronidazole, namely Flagyl tablet.

Treatment (2): using formula 3tA
A tablet containing 125 mg metronidazole with Carbopol 934 in drug: polymer ratio 2:1 w/w.

Treatment (3): using formula 5tB
A tablet containing 125 mg metronidazole with CMC in drug: polymer ratio 1:1 w/w.

Treatment (4): using formula 7tA
A tablet containing 125 mg metronidazole with methyl cellulose in drug: polymer ratio 2:1 w/w.

Treatment (5): using formula 1cC
A capsule containing 125 mg metronidazole with HPMC 15000 in drug: polymer ratio 2:3 w/w.

Treatment (6): using formula 8cD
A capsule containing 125 mg metronidazole with pectin in drug: polymer ratio 1:2 w/w.

2-Subject selection:

The subjects will be normal healthy adult male volunteers, medical staff members of El-Hussein hospital who participate in this study during their free time. Each wills discuss the clinical design and the data on metronidazole. The total number of volunteers participating in the study was six.

<u>3-Study design:</u>

The six volunteers participated in a four-way crossover study, where each study was separated from the other by an interval of at least one week. The dose of metronidazole was equivalent to 125 mg drug taken with 200 ml water after light breakfast.

The volunteers did not take any drug a week before or during the trial. Every one was supervised by a physician, who was responsible for their safety and collection of blood samples during the trial. All volunteers were fasted at least for 12 hours before administration of dose, and were canulated at start of trial following the withdrawal of 5-ml control venous blood specimen (0-hour).

<u>4-Sample collection:</u>

Venous blood samples were withdrawn via an intravenous cannula or by vein puncture on the following time schedule: 0 (pre-dose), 0.25, 0.5, 1, 2, 3, 4, 6, 12, and 24 hour post-dose of reference tablet and prepared floating dosage form of metronidazole.

<u>5-Handling of the samples:</u>

Blood samples were then centrifuged .The resulting plasma fraction was transferred by pipetting into pre-labeled polypropylene screw-cap tubes. Samples were flash frozen and then stored immediately at −20 °C.

6-Chromatographic system and Conditions:

Simple and sensitive HPLC method for determination of metronidazole in human serum has been used. The mobile phase, consisted of acetonitrile-0.01 M phosphate solution ($K_2H_2PO_4$), pH 4.7,15:85,v/v, was degassed and filtered through a 0.45 μm filter (Millipore, Sainet-Quentin, Yvelines, France). The flow rate was 1ml/minute. The detection wavelength was 324 nm. The injection volum was 20 μl and the run time was 9 minutes. The mobile phase was freshly prepared. Chromatography was carried out at ambient temperature.

7- Stock and working standard solutions:

Stock solution of metronidazole was prepared by dissolving 100mg metronidazole in 100 ml ethanol. This solution was used to prepare working standard solutions daily for different concentrations between 0.1mg/ml and 0.01μg /ml by dilution with deionized water.

8- Stock and working internal standard solution:

The internal standard solution was prepared by dissolving 100 mg tinidazole in 100 ml ethanol. The working internal standard was prepared by taking 10 ml from this solution in 100 ml ethanol (100 μg/ml).

9- Calibration curve:

Aliquots of the working standard solution of metronidazole corresponding to concentration ranged from 0.01-10 μg/ml and 50 μl of the internal standard working solution were introduced into centrifuge tubes provided with tight sealing polyethylene caps. 200 μl plasma was added to each tube to produce calibration curve samples. Table (141) and Figure (53) show the results produced.

10- Sample preparation:

In 1.5-ml glass tube, 200 µl of plasma sample was mixed with 50 µl of the ethanol containing 10 mg/100ml tinidazole as internal standard (100 µg/ ml) and 50 µl of 0.1 M ZnSO$_4$. The tubes were capped ,vortex-mixed for 15 second, and kept frozen at –20°C for 15 minutes. The tubes were then centrifuged at 1600rpm for 2 minutes. An aliquot (10 µl) of the supernatant was injected using the chromatographic conditions described before.

11- Within –Day accuracy and precision:

Plasma samples spiked with different amounts of metronidazole were analyzed three times on the same day. These results are shown in Table (142).

12-Day-to-Day accuracy and precision:

Plasma samples spiked with different amounts of metronidazole were analyzed on three different days. Table (143) demonstrates the accuracy of the method, within the concentration range of 0.01-5 µg/ml.

13- Calculation:

200 µl of the different plasma samples collected from each volunteer was treated as mentioned above. Standard curve was constructed using peak area ratios of metronidazole to the internal standard. The equation of the curve was used for calculation of unknown concentration of collected plasma samples. The equation is y=0.281 x where y is the peak area ratio (drug/internal standard) and x is metronidazole concentration µg/ml.

14- Physical Recovery:

The physical recovery of metronidazole was determined by comparing the peak area ratios measured in extracted serum samples containing known concentrations of metronidazole with those peak area ratios measured in unextracted samples containing the same concentrations of metronidazole. Recovery carried out by this method was found to be 95.2 % as average of three replicate assays with relative standard deviation (1.59).

An example of HPLC chromatogram of extract from blank human plasma (drug-free) sample and from human plasma spiked with 5 μg/ml of metronidazole and 5 μg/ml of tinidazole are illustrated in Figure (52).

Both metronidazole plasma levels determined for each subject and the mean plasma levels after administration of the investigated treatment to six human volunteers were represented in Tables (144-149), and illustrated in Figures (54-65).

The pharmacokinetic parameters and the relative bioavailability were estimated using the data obtained from plotting metronidazole plasma concentration versus time. A special computer program was used for calculating the above parameters. The data were shown in Table (150).

Table (141): Relation between metronidazole concentration (μg/ml) and peak area ratio in human plasma as determined by HPLC method.

Concentration (μg/ml)	Peak area ratio
0.00	0.000
0.01	0.0229
0.03	0.0310
0.05	0.0312
0.10	0.0923
0.50	0.2020
1.00	0.2732
2.50	0.6780
5.00	1.4088

Table (142): Within day precision of the determination of metronidazole.

Spiked conc.(μg/ml)	Peak area ratio			
	1	2	3	Mean ±SD
0.00	0.00	0.00	0.00	0.00
0.01	0.0229	0.0258	0.035	0.024±0.0015
0.03	0.031	0.04	0.031	0.034±0.005
0.05	0.0612	0.0614	0.0611	0.061±0.00015
0.10	0.0923	0.1	0.092	0.095±0.0045
0.50	0.20	0.25	0.215	0.222±0.025
1.00	0.273	0.274	0.280	0.275±0.0037
2.50	0.678	0.680	0.685	0.681±0.0035
5.00	1.4088	1.410	1.4087	1.409±0.0007
Slope	0.2807	0.2819	0.2016	0.254±0.046
correlation coefficient(r)	0.9932	0.9874	0.9924	0.991±0.003

Table (143): Day to day precision of the determination of metronidazole.

Spiked conc. (μg/ml)	Peak area ratio after (day)			
	1	2	3	Mean ±SD
0.00	0.00	0.00	0.00	0.00
0.01	0.0229	0.04	0.035	0.033±0.0087
0.03	0.031	0.025	0.037	0.031±0.006
0.05	0.0612	0.0625	0.061	0.064±0.0047
0.10	0.0923	0.0931	0.0923	0.098±0.01
0.50	0.020	0.0200	0.0215	0.227±0.025
1.00	0.273	0.273	0.2781	0.275±0.0029
2.50	0.678	0.680	0.782	0.71±0.0059
5.00	1.4088	1.400	1.415	1.41±0.007
Slope	0.2807	0.2802	0.2903	0.284±0.0056
correlation coefficient (r)	0.9932	0.9877	0.9869	0.989±0.0034

Table (144): Metronidazole plasma concentration after oral tablet administration of treatment No. I (commercial metronidazole tablet) to six human volunteers.

Time (hr)	Plasma concentration (µg/ml) of metronidazole						Mean plasma conc. (ug/ml)±SD
	H1	H2	H3	H4	H5	H6	
0.00	0.00	0.00	0.00	0.00	0.00	0.00	0.00
0.25	1.41	1.45	1.43	1.4	1.44	1.44	1.43±0.019408
0.50	4.4	4.3	4.05	4.2	4	4.6	4.30±0.216025
1.00	5.4	5.30	5.5	5.3	5	5	5.30±0.207364
2.00	5.08	5.17	5.1	5.00	4.99	5.17	5.08±0.078677
3.00	4.9	5.11	5.00	4.27	4.4	5.01	4.27±0.253298
4.00	4.2	3.89	3.70	4.11	3.9	3.95	3.70±0.123518
6.00	3.5	3.75	3.45	3.4	3.37	3.25	3.45±0.168127
8.00	2.98	2.57	2.88	2.81	2.78	2.7	2.78±0.14222
12.0	2.57	2.38	2.51	2.61	2.43	2.47	2.51±0.086197
24.0	1.20	1.21	1.35	1.26	1.01	1.119	1.20±0.116985

H: human volunteer.

Table (145): Metronidazole plasma concentration after oral tablet administration of treatment No. II containing drug: Carbopol (2:1) to six human volunteers.

Time (hr)	Plasma concentration (μg/ml) of metronidazole						Mean plasma conc.(ug/ml)±SD
	H1	H2	H3	H4	H5	H6	
0.00	0.00	0.00	0.00	0.00	0.00	0.00	0.00
0.25	0.825	0.845	0.835	0.801	0.811	0.833	0.825±0.01634
0.50	0.98	1.00	0.96	0.97	1.02	1.12	1.00±0.058793
1.00	1.115	1.23	1.31	1.25	1.24	1.22	1.22±0.063541
2.00	1.425	1.489	1.6	1.71	1.225	1.101	1.425±0.22843
3.00	1.214	1.736	1.495	1.431	1.32	1.401	1.43±0.177432
4.00	2.098	2.10	2.11	1.92	2.16	2.20	2.098±0.09600
6.00	1.76	1.673	1.7	1.65	1.645	1.61	1.673±0.05211
8.00	1.378	1.421	1.355	1.393	1.415	1.401	1.393±0.02448
12.0	1.04	0.632	0.822	0.545	0.895	0.997	0.822±0.19814
24.0	0.335	0.385	0.188	0.269	0.201	0.235	0.269±0.07765

H: human volunteer.

Table (146): Metronidazole plasma concentration after oral tablet administration of treatment No. III containing drug: CMC (1:1) to six human volunteers.

Time (hr)	Plasma concentration (μg/ml) of metronidazole						Mean plasma conc.(ug/ml)± SD
	H1	H2	H3	H4	H5	H6	
0.00	0.00	0.00	0.00	0.00	0.00	0.00	0.00
0.25	1.117	1.11	1.123	1.12	1.113	1.121	1.117±0.00500
0.50	1.329	1.678	1.437	1.53	1.701	1.523	1.533±0.14155
1.00	1.533	1.501	1.517	1.515	1.511	1.529	1.517±0.01177
2.00	1.471	1.488	1.473	1.455	1.467	1.478	1.472±0.01102
3.00	1.39	1.415	1.42	1.413	1.411	1.431	1.413±0.01348
4.00	1.385	1.458	1.404	1.351	1.298	1.53	1.404±0.08148
6.00	1.272	1.25	1.231	1.257	1.287	1.25	1.257±0.01946
8.00	1.1	1.302	1.258	1.341	1.229	1.15	1.23±0.091203
12.0	1.335	1.201	1.28	1.42	1.19	1.23	1.276±0.08873
24.0	1.14	1.257	1.37	1.31	1.27	1.2	1.257±0.08084

H: human volunteer.

Table (147): Metronidazole plasma concentration after oral tablet administration of treatment No. IV containing drug: methyl cellulose (2:1) to six human volunteers.

Time (hr)	Plasma concentration (µg/ml) of metronidazole						Mean plasma conc.(ug/ml)±SD
	H1	H2	H3	H4	H5	H6	
0.00	0.00	0.00	0.00	0.00	0.00	0.00	0.00
0.25	0.822	0.915	0.880	0.795	0.690	0.820	0.82±0.822
0.50	1.270	1.250	1.310	1.210	1.201	1.30	1.25±0.0452
1.00	1.402	1.431	1.419	1.42	1.428	1.411	1.4185±0.01074
2.00	1.554	1.575	1.567	1.558	1.531	1.560	1.558±0.01495
3.00	1.371	1.37	1.32	1.25	1.20	1.40	1.32±0.07847
4.00	1.20	1.126	1.19	1.11	1.02	1.115	1.126±0.065086
6.00	0.967	1.01	0.937	0.887	0.921	0.9	0.937±0.045506
8.00	1.487	1.501	1.481	1.493	1.49	1.50	1.492±0.007694
12.0	1.243	1.263	1.223	1.25	1.246	1.255	1.246±0.013574
24.0	1.351	1.423	1.328	1.31	1.305	1.255	1.328±0.056095

H: human volunteer.

Table (148): Metronidazole plasma concentration after oral capsule administration of treatment No. V containing drug: HPMC 15000 (2:3) to six human volunteers.

Time (hr)	Plasma concentration (µg/ml) of metronidazole						Mean plasma conc.(ug/ml)±SD
	H1	H2	H3	H4	H5	H6	
0.00	0.00	0.00	0.00	0.00	0.00	0.00	0.00
0.25	0.115	0.125	0.123	0.117	0.11	0.101	0.115±0.008819
0.50	0.14	0.107	0.08	0.093	0.127	0.10	0.107±0.022176
1.00	0.191	0.23	0.198	0.157	0.29	0.127	0.198±0.057017
2.00	0.341	0.355	0.37	0.354	0.335	0.374	0.354±0.015381
3.00	0.4115	0.42	0.415	0.40	0.407	0.391	0.407±0.010557
4.00	0.378	0.369	0.381	0.36	0.365	0.358	0.369±0.009397
6.00	0.332	0.34	0.35	0.339	0.357	0.343	0.343±0.008826
8.00	0.288	0.311	0.301	0.309	0.315	0.281	0.301±0.01363
12.0	0.199	0.216	0.234	0.231	0.233	0.188	0.216±0.019529
24.0	0.12	0.04	0.08	0.066	0.031	0.059	0.066±0.031818

H: human volunteer.

Table (149): Metronidazole plasma concentration after oral capsule administration of treatment No. VI containing drug: pectin (1:2) to six human volunteers.

Time (hr)	Plasma concentration (μg/ml) of metronidazole						Mean plasma conc.(ug/ml)±SD
	H1	H2	H3	H4	H5	H6	
0.00	0.00	0.00	0.00	0.00	0.00	0.00	0.00
0.25	0.017	0.033	0.055	0.059	0.011	0.023	0.033±0.02
0.50	0.158	0.301	0.235	0.171	0.37	0.18	0.235±0.084412
1.00	0.235	0.345	0.241	0.235	0.157	0.2	0.235±0.62359
2.00	0.45	0.466	0.471	0.439	0.454	0.441	0.454±0.12973
3.00	0.511	0.498	0.5	0.501	0.515	0.52	0.508±0.009094
4.00	0.508	0.521	0.488	0.493	0.515	0.525	0.508±0.015042
6.00	0.399	0.488	0.375	0.428	0.435	0.444	0.428±0.038871
8.00	0.336	0.346	0.33	0.327	0.32	0.354	0.336±0.012613
12.0	0.285	0.271	0.28	0.266	0.258	0.267	0.271±0.009867
24.0	0.0887	0.098	0.123	0.14	0.154	0.135	0.123±0.02528

H: human volunteer.

Table (150): Pharmacokinetic parameters of different metronidazole treatments administered orally to human volunteers.

Formula Parameter	Treatment I	Treatment II	Treatment III	Treatment IV	Treatment V	Treatment VI
Dose(mg)	250	125	125	125	125	125
$C_{max}(\mu g/ml)$	5.3	2.098	1.53	1.558	0.407	0.508
$t_{max}(hr)$	1	4	1	2	3	3
$K_{ab}(hr^{-1})$	10.21531	0.595565	1.099681	0.165768	0.725723	0.4249
$t_{1/2ab}(hr)$	0.067839	1.163601	0.630183	4.180536	0.954909	1.6332
$K_{el}(hr^{-1})$	0.060953	0.101715	0.005884	0.111016	0.08875	0.066767
$t_{1/2el}(hr)$	11.36941	6.813172	117.7814	6.242326	7.808489	10.37945
$V_d(L)$	49.73128	49.88064	90.09014	209.4549	245.5981	178.1335
TCR(ml/min)	50.2121	84.55993	8.834508	387.5486	363.2787	198.2226
$AUC_{0-24}(\mu g.hr/ml)$	63.365	23.21425	30.96575	30.5945	5.244875	6.766625
$AUC_{24-\infty}(\mu g.hr/ml)$	19.68729	2.644651	213.6382	11.96221	0.743666	1.84224
$AUC_{0-\infty}(\mu g.hr/ml)$	83.05229	25.8589	244.604	42.55671	5.988541	8.608865
$AUMC_{0-24}(\mu g.hr^2/ml)$	571.9206	192.0411	365.5714	373.106	45.89875	62.63038
$AUMC_{24-\infty}(\mu g.hr^2/ml)$	472.4949	63.47163	5127.317	287.0929	17.84797	44.21376
$AUMC_{0-\infty}(\mu g.hr^2/ml)$	1044.416	255.5127	5492.888	660.1989	63.74672	106.8441
MRT(hr)	12.5754	9.881034	22.45625	15.51339	10.64478	12.41094
$C_{max}/AUC_{(0-24)}(hr^{-1})$	0.083642	0.090376	0.049409	0.050924	0.0776	0.075074
RB %	--	3.27	97.73	96.56	16.55	21.357

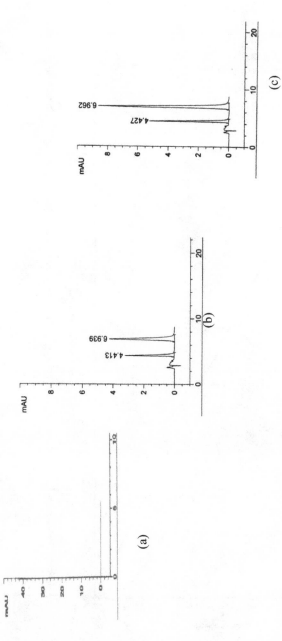

Figure (52): Chromatogram of blank human plasma (a), typical chromatograms of human plasma spiked with 5µg/ml metronidazole at 4.4 min and 5µg/ml tinidazole (internal standard) at 6.9 min (b), as well as the chromatograms of plasma sample obtained from a volunteer after oral administration of formula 3tA Figure (c).

344

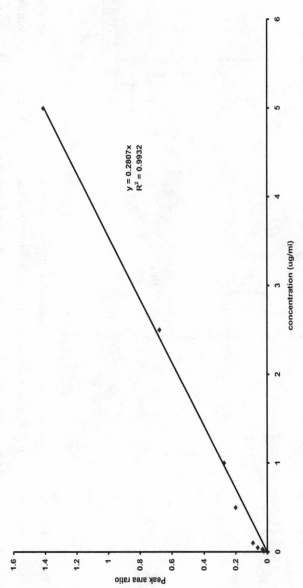

$y = 0.2807x$
$R^2 = 0.9932$

Figure (53): HPLC standard calibration curve of metronidazole in human plasma using tinidazole as internal standard.

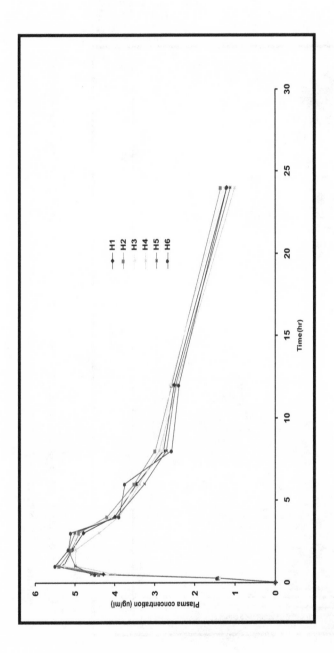

Figure (54): Metronidazole plasma concentration-time curve after oral dose of commercial metronidazole tablet (treatment I) to six human volunteers.

346

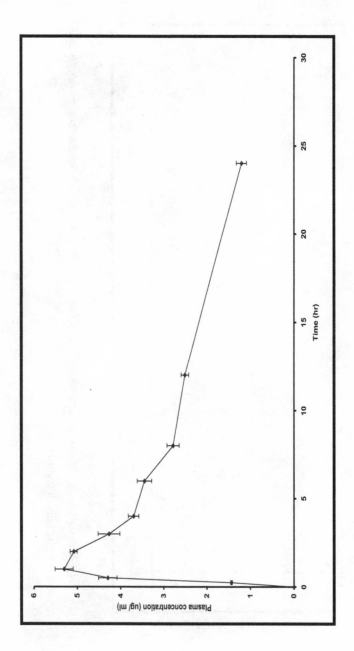

Figure (55): Metronidazole mean plasma concentration-time curve after oral dose of commercial metronidazole tablet (treatment I) to six human volunteers.

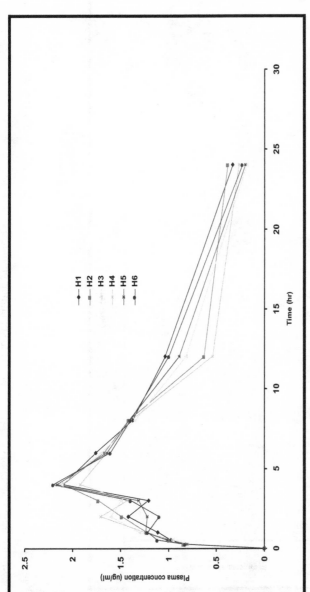

Figure (56): Metronidazole plasma concentration-time curve after oral dose of metronidazole tablet containing drug: Carbopol (2:1)(treatment II) to six human volunteers.

348

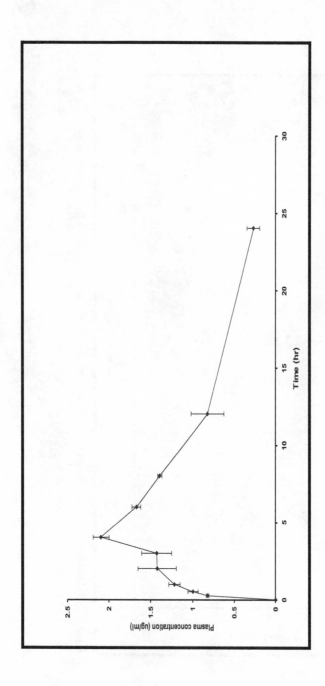

Figure (57): Metronidazole mean plasma concentration-time curve after oral dose of metronidazole tablet containing drug: Carbopol (2:1) (treatment II) to six human volunteers.

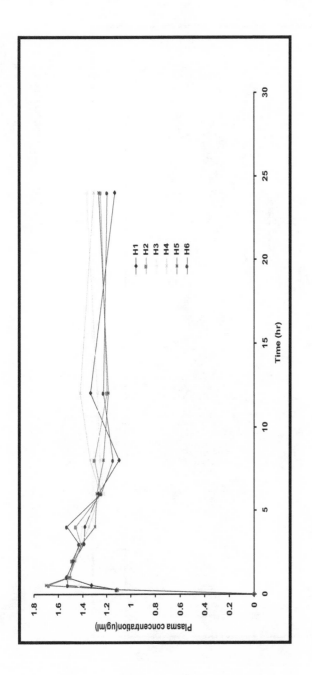

Figure (58): Metronidazole plasma concentration-time curve after oral dose of metronidazole tablet containing drug: CMC (1:1) (treatment III)to six human volunteers.

350

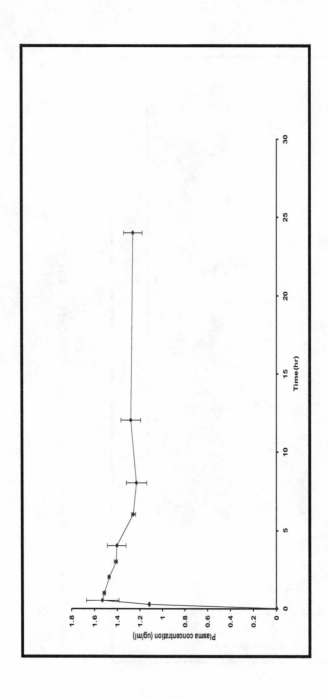

Figure (59): Metronidazole mean plasma concentration-time curve after oral dose of metronidazole tablet containing drug: CMC (1:1) (treatment III) to six human volunteers.

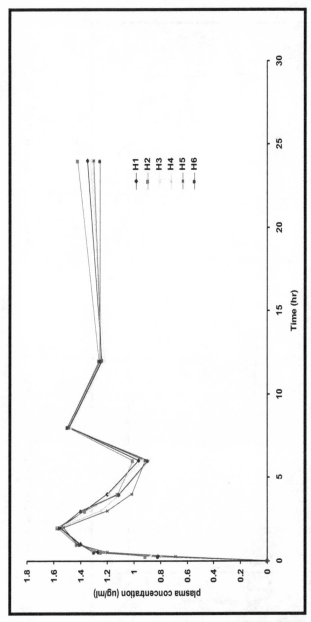

Figure (60): Metronidazole plasma concentration-time curve after oral dose of metronidazole tablet containing drug: methyl cellulose (2:1)(treatment IV) to six human volunteers.

352

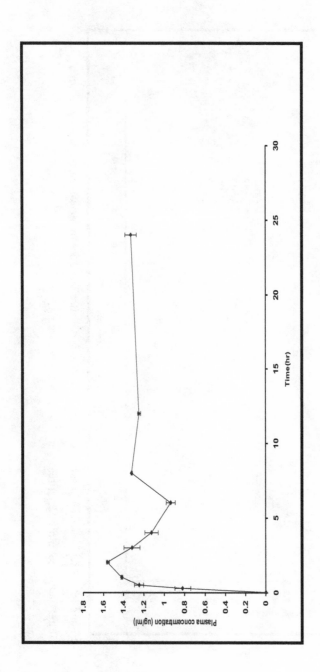

Figure (61): Metronidazole plasma concentration-time curve after oral dose of metronidazole tablet containing drug: methyl cellulose (2:1)(treatment IV) to six human volunteers.

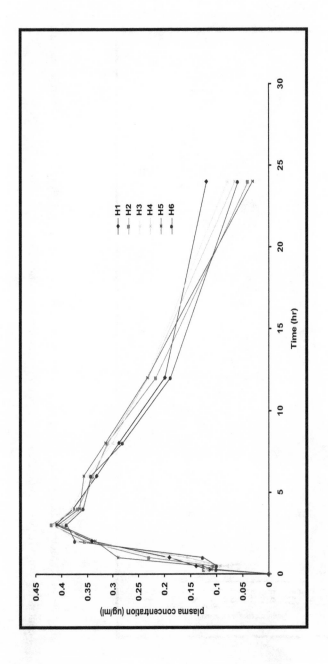

Figure (62): Metronidazole plasma concentration-time curve after oral dose of metronidazole capsule containing drug: HPMC 15000(2:3) (treatment V) to six human volunteers.

354

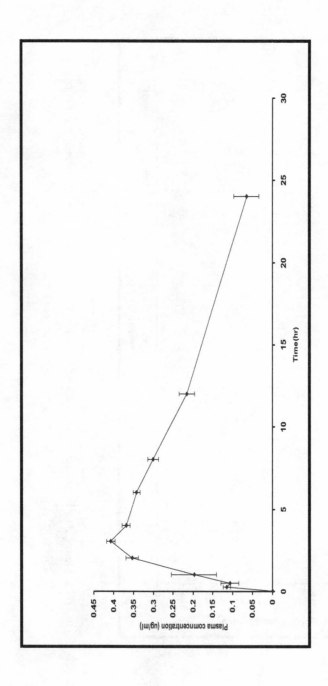

Figure (63): Metronidazole mean plasma concentration-time curve after oral dose of metronidazole capsule containing drug: HPMC 15000(2:3) (treatment V) to six human volunteers.

355

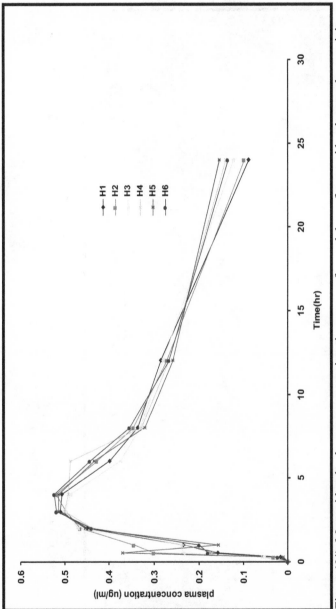

Figure (64): Metronidazole plasma concentration-time curve after oral dose of metronidazole capsule containing drug: pectin (1:2) (treatment VI)to six human volunteers.

356

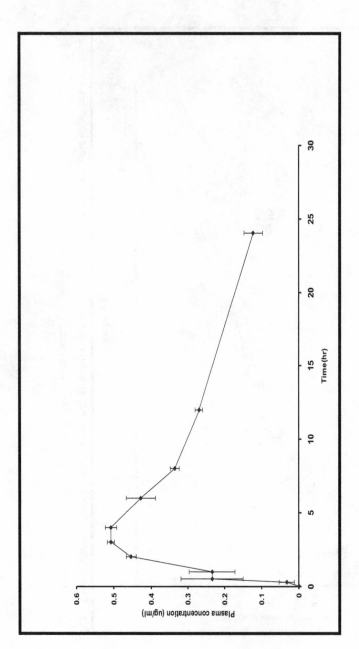

Figure (65): Metronidazole mean plasma concentration-time curve after oral dose of metronidazole capsule containing drug: pectin (1:2) (treatment VI) to six human volunteers.

Results and Discussion

The bioequivalence of the controlled release floating metronidazole dosage forms; in relation to that available in the market was determined in human volunteers. The tested formulae and the commercial product were administered to six human volunteers. The plasma was then collected, and t_{max}, C_{max}, AUC $_{0-\infty}$, $AUMC_{0-\infty}$ and MRT were used for assessing the bioavailability of metronidazole product under investigation.

A new technique was specially developed for this assay, where the method of (Jensen and Gugler, 1983) was adopted. The HPLC conditions for separation of metronidazole such as the mobile phase composition, the type of column and its dimension, wavelength of the detection were investigated. C_8 and C_{18} columns of different dimensions and particle sizes were used. It was found that C_{18} column (30 cm × 3.9 mm) with average particle size 10 μm give the best suitable resolution. The mobile phase composition was prepared with either 0.005 M KH_2PO_4 (pH 4.5)-methanol-tetrahydrofuran in ratio 82.6:16.5:0.9 or with 0.01 M KH_2PO_4 (pH 4.7)-acetonitrile in ratio 85:15 v/v. It was shown that the best resolution of metronidazole was achieved with a mobile phase 0.01M KH_2PO_4-acetonitrile (85:15 v/v) at flow rate 1 ml/minute.

In an attempt to increase the sensitivity of the assay, different wavelengths, 318, 324, and 254 nm for detection of both metronidazole and tinidazole (as internal standard) were utilized. The highest sensitivity was accomplished at 324 nm.

358

The described method utilizes no organic extraction as do the GLC and TLC methods (Midha, et al., 1973; Bergan and Arnold, 1980; Gattavecchia et al., 1981) and one of the HPLC methods (Lanbeck and Lindstrom, 1979).The previously described HPLC methods used no internal standard, the use of which increase accuracy (Nilsson-Ehle et al., 1981; Wheeler et al., 19878; Marques et al, 1978). In addition protein precipitation was reported to be a problem if samples were left standing for long periods of time, as would be the case when automatic injectors are used (Wheeler et al 1978). The use of $ZnSO_4$ and cooling step described here has eliminated this problem, with no additional precipitation being seen over 6 hours. Also, by not using perchloric acid (Nilsson-Ehle et al, 1981) or trichloroacetic acid for protein precipitation, column life is greatly extended.

A typical chromatogram for 200 μl of blank human plasma is shown in Figure (52a).There was no components that elute with metronidazole or tinidazole.

Figure (52b) shows the typical chromatograms of plasma spiked with 5μg/ml metronidazole and 5μg/ml tinidazole (internal standard), as well as the chromatogram of plasma sample obtained from a volunteers after oral administration of formula 3tA Figure (52c).

Metronidazole and tinidazole were well resolved and the retention times were 4.4 and 6.9 minutes, respectively. No interfering peaks were observed in the chromatogram of the blank human serum. Tinidazole is a good choice as internal standard due to its reasonable retention time and similar spectral properties to metronidazole.

Table (141) illustrates the peak area ratios and concentrations of metronidazole in μg/ml measured in human plasma by the sensitive HPLC method. Figure (53) shows a plot of metronidazole concentration in μg/ml in control human plasma versus peak area ratio. Linear regression analysis was used to calculate the slope, intercept, and correlation coefficient (r) of the calibration line. The linearity found to be quite satisfactory and reproducible with time. The equation of linear regression was y = 0.2807x for metronidazole concentration ranging from 0.01 to 5 μg/ml. The correlation coefficient(r) of the line was 0.9932 and the percentage recovery was (95.2%). From the table, it was found that the straight line obtained passed through the origin which verify and obey Beer's Lambert law.

The day to day reproducibility of the assay for plasma samples was evaluated from spiked plasma standards at three times in the same day (Table 142) and at three different days (Table 143). The average correlation coefficient was 0.991 and 0.989, respectively. These results confirmed excellent linearity of the calibration lines and high reproducibility of the assay.

For comparison of the commercial metronidazole tablets (namely flagyl) versus the chosen prepared floating dosage forms of metronidazole (formulae 3tA, 5tB, 7tA, 1cC, and 8cD), plasma concentrations of metronidazole after administration of both flagyl and the tested formulae in six human volunteers were investigated.

Table (144) and figure (55) show the time course of mean human plasma concentrations of metronidazole after oral administration of flagyl

360

tablets to six human volunteers. A rapid rise in the plasma metronidazole concentration after dosing with the flagyl tablet within first hour was observed. The flagyl tablets show mean peak plasma concentration of 5.3 µg/ml and was reached after 1 hour.

These results are in agreement with the reported C_{max}, t_{max} of metronidazole orally administered, which is 5 µg/ml achieved in average 1 to 2 hours after 250 mg oral dose (Martindale, 1993; Fredercisson et al., 1987; Ralph et al.,1974).

The pharmacokinetic parameters (k_{ab}, k_{el}, $t_{1/2ab}$, and $t_{1/2\ el}$) for commercial metronidazole tablet (flagyl), were calculated from the curve representing the relation between plasma concentration and time. The residual method for this calculation has been used, and the data were represented in Table (150).

The k_{ab} (the first order absorption rate constant) of metronidazole after dosing of its commercial tablets (flagyl) to six human volunteers found to be 10.21531 hr^{-1}.While the $t_{1/2\ ab}$ of the same product has the mean value of 0.067839 hr.

The mean value of k_{el} of metronidazole after oral administration of commercial metronidazole tablets (flagyl) to six human volunteers was found to be 0.060953 hr^{-1}. In addition the elimination half-life ($t_{1/2\ el}$) of the same product was found to be 11.36941 hour.

The mean value of $AUC_{0-\infty}$ which reflects the total amount of active drug which reaches the systemic circulation was found to be 83.05229 µg.hr/ml. While the mean value of $AUMC_{0-\infty}$ was found to be 1044.416 µg.hr^2/ml, so the MRT which is the mean residence time of metronidazole in the body was calculated from the ratio of $AUMC_{0-\infty}$ to $AUC_{0-\infty}$ and was found to be 12.5754 hour. These data were represented in Table (150).

The total clearance rate (TCR) of metronidazole after dosing of its commercial tablets (flagyl) was found to be 50.52121 ml/min.

The apparent volume of distribution (V_d) of metronidazole following the administration of its commercial tablets (flagyl) was 49.73128 liters. This determined value of V_d is in a good harmony with previously determined range 0.25-0.85 liters/kg (Bennett et al., 1994, Eradiri et al., 1988).

The mean of C_{max}/AUC_{0-24} which is a measure used to evaluate the absorption of the estimated formula, was calculated for metronidazole after oral administration of its commercial tablets (flagyl) and found to be 0.083642 hr^{-1}.

The time course of metronidazole in human plasma after oral administration of treatment II (metronidazole tablets containing Carbopol 934 in drug: polymer ratio 2:1), treatment III (metronidazole tablet containing CMC in drug: polymer ratio 1:1), treatment IV (metronidazole tablet containing methyl cellulose in drug: polymer ratio 2:1), treatment V

362

(metronidazole capsule containing HPMC 15000 in drug: polymer ratio 2:3), and treatment VI (metronidazole capsule containing pectin in drug: polymer ratio 1:2), and their pharmacokinetics indices are shown in Tables 144 to 150 and Figures 56 to 65.

It is obvious that, the mean plasma peak concentration (C_{max}) of metronidazole after oral administration of the investigated formulae was found to be 2.098, 1.53, 1.558, 0.407, and 0.508µg/ml, while T_{max} reached at 4, 1, 2, 3, and 3 hours after administration of treatment II (metronidazole tablets containing Carbopol 934 in drug: polymer ratio 2:1), treatment III (metronidazole tablet containing CMC in drug: polymer ratio 1:1), treatment IV (metronidazole tablet containing methyl cellulose in drug: polymer ratio 2:1), treatment V(metronidazole capsule containing HPMC 15000 in drug: polymer ratio 2:3), and treatment VI (metronidazole capsule containing pectin in drug: polymer ratio 1:2), respectively.

Thus the investigated treatments can be arranged in descending manner, regarding the metronidazole peak plasma concentration (C_{max}) after being orally administered to six human volunteers, as follows: metronidazole tablet containing Carbopol 934 with drug: polymer ratio 2:1 (treatment II), metronidazole tablet containing methyl cellulose with drug: polymer ratio 2:1 (treatment IV), metronidazole tablet containing CMC with drug: polymer ratio 1:1 (treatment III), metronidazole capsule containing pectin with drug: polymer ratio 1:2 (treatment VI), and metronidazole capsule containing HPMC 15000 with drug: polymer ratio 2:3 (treatment V), and. In other terms, metronidazole tablets containing Carbopol 934 with drug: polymer ratio 2:1 (treatment II) has the highest rate and extent of drug absorption concerning oral treatments estimated.

A summary of the pharmacokinetic parameters for the tested dosage forms of metronidazole after being orally administered to six human volunteers were shown in Table (150). These parameters were done using residual method (Shargel et al., 1993).

Regarding the amount of metronidazole absorbed and reached the circulation ($AUC_{0-\infty}$) after oral administration of metronidazole tablets containing Carbopol 934 with drug: polymer ratio 2:1 (treatment II), metronidazole tablets containing CMC in drug: polymer ratio 1:1 (treatment III), metronidazole tablets containing methyl cellulose in drug: polymer ratio 2:1 (treatment IV), metronidazole capsules containing HPMC 15000 in drug: polymer ratio 2:3 (treatment V), and metronidazole capsules containing pectin in drug: polymer ratio 1:2 (treatment VI), were found to be 25.8589, 244.604, 42.5567, 5.988541, and 8.608865 µg.hr/ml, respectively.

On the other hand, $AUMC_{0-\infty}$ which is the area under the first moment time curve for metronidazole after oral dosing of metronidazole tablets prepared with Carbopol 934 in drug: polymer ratio 2:1 (treatment II), metronidazole tablets prepared with CMC in drug: polymer ratio 1:1 (treatment III), metronidazole tablets prepared with methyl cellulose in drug: polymer ratio 2:1 (treatment IV), metronidazole capsules prepared with HPMC 15000 in drug: polymer ratio 2:3 (treatment V), and metronidazole capsules prepared with pectin in drug: polymer ratio 1:2 (treatment VI),show a mean value of 255.5127, 5492.888, 660.1989, 63.74672, and 106.8441 µg.hr^2/ml, respectively.

The mean residence time values of metronidazole in the body (MRT) after oral administration of investigated formulae were found to be 9.881034, 22.45625, 15.51339, 10.64478, and 12.41094 hours concerning metronidazole tablets containing Carbopol 934 with drug: polymer ratio 2:1 (treatment II), metronidazole tablets containing CMC in drug: polymer ratio 1:1 (treatment III), metronidazole tablets containing methyl cellulose in drug: polymer ratio 2:1 (treatment IV), metronidazole capsules containing HPMC 15000 in drug: polymer ratio 2:3 (treatment V), and metronidazole capsules containing pectin in drug: polymer ratio 1:2 (treatment VI), respectively.

The absorption rate constant K_{ab} values of metronidazole following oral administration of the investigated prepared formulae were found to be 0.595565, 1.099681, 0.165768, 0.725723, and 0.42429 hr^{-1}concerning treatment II (metronidazole tablet containing Carbopol 934 in drug: polymer ratio 2:1), treatment III (metronidazole tablet containing CMC in drug: polymer ratio 1:1), treatment IV (metronidazole tablet containing methyl cellulose in drug: polymer ratio 2:1), treatment V (metronidazole capsule containing HPMC 15000 in drug: polymer ratio 2:3), and treatment VI (metronidazole capsule containing pectin in ratio 1:2), respectively. While their $t_{1/2\ ab}$ values which can be determined from the equation $t_{1/2} = 0.639/K_{ab}$ were found to be 1.16360, 0.630183, 4.180536, 7.808489, and 1.63332 hour, respectively.

Regarding the K_{ab} of the previous metronidazole tablets and capsules, one can arrange the investigated treatments, in descending manner, as follows: metronidazole tablets containing CMC in ratio 1:1 (treatment III), metronidazole capsule containing HPMC 15000 in ratio 2:3 (treatment V), metronidazole tablets containing Carbopol 934 in ratio 2:1 (treatment II), metronidazole capsules containing pectin in ratio 1:2 (treatment VI), and metronidazole tablets containing methyl cellulose in ratio 2:1 (treatment IV).

Concerning the k_{el} of treatment II (metronidazole tablet containing Carbopol 934 in ratio 2:1), treatment III (metronidazole tablet containing CMC in ratio 1:1), treatment IV (metronidazole tablet containing methyl cellulose in ratio 2:1), treatment V (metronidazole capsule containing HPMC 15000 in ratio 2:3), and treatment VI (metronidazole capsule containing pectin in ratio 1:2) was found to be 0.101715, 0.005884, 0.111016, 0.08875, and 0.066767 hr^{-1}, respectively. In addition, their t $_{\frac{1}{2} \, el}$ show a mean values of 6.813172, 117.7814, 6.24326, 7.80849, and 10.37945 hour, respectively.

With reference to k_{el} of the metronidazole tablets and capsules employed, one can be arranged for the investigated treatmens,in descending manner, as follows: metronidazole tablets containing methyl cellulose with drug: polymer ratio 2:1 (treatment IV), metronidazole tablets containing Carbopol 934 with drug: polymer ratio 2:1 (treatment II), metronidazole capsules containing HPMC 15000 with drug: polymer ratio 2:3 (treatment V), metronidazole capsules containing pectin with drug: polymer ratio 1:2 (treatment VI), and metronidazole tablets containing CMC with drug: polymer ratio 1:1 (treatment III) .

The total clearance rate (TCR) of metronidazole after administration of investigated treatments was found to be 84.55993 ml/min for metronidazole tablet containing Carbopol 934 in drug: polymer ratio 2:1 (treatment II),8.834508 ml/min for metronidazole tablet containing CMC in drug: polymer ratio 1:1 (treatment III), 387.5486 ml/min for metronidazole tablet containing methyl cellulose in drug: polymer ratio 2:1 (treatment IV), 363.2787 ml/min for metronidazole capsules containing HPMC 15000 in drug: polymer ratio 2:3 (treatment V), and 198.2226 ml/min for metronidazole capsules containing pectin in drug: polymer ratio 1:2 (treatment VI).

The apparent volume of distribution (Vd) of metronidazole after oral dose administration of investigated formulae showed a values of 49.88064, 90.09014, 209.4549, 245.5981, and 178.1335 liters concerning metronidazole tablets containing Carbopol 934 with drug: polymer ratio 2:1 (treatment II), metronidazole tablets containing CMC in drug: polymer ratio 1:1 (treatment III), metronidazole tablets containing methyl cellulose in drug: polymer ratio 2:1 (treatment IV), metronidazole capsules containing HPMC 15000 in drug: polymer ratio 2:3 (treatment V), and metronidazole capsules containing pectin in drug: polymer ratio 1:2 (treatment VI), respectively.

The mean C_{max}/AUC_{0-24} was calculated and found to be 0.090376, 0.049409, 0.050924, 0.0776, 0.075074hr^{-1} concerning treatment II (metronidazole tablets containing Carbopol 934 in drug: polymer ratio 2:1), treatment III (metronidazole tablets containing CMC in drug: polymer ratio 1:1), treatment IV (metronidazole tablets containing methyl cellulose in drug: polymer ratio 2:1), treatment V (metronidazole capsules containing HPMC 15000 in drug: polymer ratio 2:3), and treatment VI (metronidazole capsules containing pectin in drug: polymer ratio 1:2), respectively.

Regarding the mean C_{max}/AUC_{0-24}, one can arrange the investigated treatments, descendingly, as follows: metronidazole tablets containing Carbopol 934 in drug: polymer ratio 2:1 (treatment II), metronidazole capsules containing HPMC 15000 in drug: polymer ratio 2:3 (treatment V), metronidazole capsules containing pectin in drug: polymer ratio 1:2 (treatment VI), metronidazole tablets containing methyl cellulose in drug: polymer ratio 2:1 (treatment IV), and metronidazole tablets containing CMC in drug: polymer ratio 1:1 (treatment III).

Relative (apparent) availability is the availability of the drug from a drug product as compared to a recognized standard (Shargel et al., 1993)

The relative bioavailability of metronidazole tablets and capsules to standard commercial tablets naming flagyl can be determined for the tested formulae based on AUC $_{0-24}$. The relative bioavailability % was found to be 73.27% for metronidazole tablets containing Carbopol 934 in ratio 2:1 (treatment II), 97.73 % for metronidazole tablets containing CMC in drug: polymer ratio 1:1 (treatment III), 96.56% for metronidazole tablets containing methyl cellulose in drug: polymer ratio 2:1(treatment IV), 16.55% for metronidazole capsules containing HPMC 15000 in drug: polymer ratio 2:3 (treatment V), and 21.357% for metronidazole capsules containing pectin in drug: polymer ratio 1:2 (treatment VI).

368

As regards to the bioavailability of metronidazole tablets and capsules to standard commercial metronidazole tablets (flagyl),one can arrange the investigated treatments in descending manner as follows: metronidazole tablets containing CMC in drug: polymer ratio 1:1(treatment III), metronidazole tablets containing methyl cellulose in drug: polymer ratio 2:1 (treatment IV), metronidazole tablets containing Carbopol 934 in drug: polymer ratio 2:1 (treatment II), metronidazole capsules containing pectin in drug: polymer ratio 1:2 (treatment VI), and metronidazole capsules containing HPMC 15000 in drug: polymer ratio 2:3 (treatment V).

Though, the selected metronidazole tablets and capsules formulae can be ranked with respect to the mean plasma peak concentrastion (C_{max}), descindingly as follows: metronidazole tablet containing Carbopol 934 with drug: polymer ratio 2:1 (treatment II), metronidazole tablet containing methyl cellulose with drug: polymer ratio 2:1 (treatment IV), metronidazole tablet containing CMC with drug: polymer ratio 1:1 (treatment III), metronidazole capsule containing pectin with drug: polymer ratio 1:2 (treatment VI), and metronidazole capsule containing HPMC 15000 with drug: polymer ratio 2:3(treatment V).

Treatment III which is metronidazole tablets containing CMC in drug: polymer ratio 1:1 was found to be the best studied treatment as it showed short t $_{max}$, medium C $_{max}$, medium MRT, good K $_{ab}$, and the best relative bioavailability.

Conclusion

Based on the bioavailability and the pharmacokinetic data generated from the concentration/ time profiles of the investigated treatments after being orally administered to human volunteers, one can concluded the following:

1-Regarding the peak drug plasma concentration, C_{max}, the investigated treatments can be arranged, in descending manner, as follows: metronidazole tablet containing Carbopol 934 with drug: polymer ratio 2:1 (treatment II), metronidazole tablet containing methyl cellulose with drug: polymer ratio 2:1 (treatment IV), metronidazole tablet containing CMC with drug: polymer ratio 1:1 (treatment III), metronidazole capsule containing pectin with drug: polymer ratio 1:2 (treatment VI), and metronidazole capsule containing HPMC 15000 with drug: polymer ratio 2:3 (treatment V).

2-The time necessary to reach a maximum peak concentration t_{max}, which reflects the rate of drug absorption, was found to be 4 hours for metronidazole tablet containing Carbopol 934 in drug: polymer ratio 2:1, one hour for metronidazole tablet containing CMC in drug: polymer ratio 1:1, 2 hours for metronidazole tablets prepared with methyl cellulose in drug: polymer ratio 2:1, 3 hours for both metronidazole capsule containing HPMC 15000 in drug: polymer ratio 2:3and metronidazole capsule containing pectin in drug: polymer ratio 1:2.

3-The maximum $AUC_{0-\infty}$ has been showed with treatment II (metronidazole tablets containing CMC in drug: polymer ratio 1:1) and was 244.604 μg.hr/ml, while the minimum $AUC_{0-\infty}$ was belonging to treatment V (capsules containing HPMC 15000 in drug: polymer ratio 2:3) and was 5.988541 µg.hr/ml.

4-Regarding the area under plasma concentration time curve, $AUC_{0-\infty}$, which reflects the bioavailability, the investigated treatments can be arranged, in descending manner, as follows: metronidazole tablets containing CMC in drug: polymer ratio 1:1, metronidazole tablets containing methyl cellulose in drug: polymer ratio 2:1, metronidazole tablets containing Carbopol 934 with drug: polymer ratio 2:1, metronidazole capsules containing HPMC 15000 in drug: polymer ratio 2:3, and metronidazole capsules containing pectin in drug: polymer ratio 1:2.

5-Regarding the mean residence time of the investigated formulae, MRT, they can be arranged in descending manner, as follows: metronidazole tablets containing CMC in drug: polymer ratio 1:1, metronidazole tablets containing methyl cellulose in drug: polymer ratio 2:1 , metronidazole capsules containing pectin in drug: polymer ratio 1:2, metronidazole capsules containing HPMC 15000 in drug: polymer ratio 2:3 and metronidazole tablets containing Carbopol 934 with drug: polymer ratio 2:1.

6-According to the absorption rate constant, K_{ab}, the investigated treatments can be arranged, in descending order, as following: metronidazole tablets containing CMC in drug: polymer ratio 1:1 (treatment III), metronidazole capsule containing HPMC 15000 in drug: polymer ratio 2:3 (treatment V), metronidazole tablets containing Carbopol 934 in drug: polymer ratio 2:1 (treatment II), metronidazole capsules containing pectin in drug: polymer ratio 1:2 (treatment VI), and metronidazole tablets containing methyl cellulose in drug: polymer ratio 2:1 (treatment IV).

7-The elimination rate constant, k_{el}, of the investigated treatments can be arranged, in descending order, as follows: metronidazole tablets containing methyl cellulose with drug: polymer ratio 2:1 (treatment IV), metronidazole tablets containing Carbopol 934 with drug: polymer ratio 2:1 (treatment II), metronidazole capsules containing HPMC 15000 with drug: polymer ratio 2:3 (treatment V), metronidazole capsules containing pectin with drug: polymer ratio 1:2 (treatment VI), and metronidazole tablets containing CMC with drug: polymer ratio 1:1 (treatment III).

8-Regarding the percentage relative bioavailability of metronidazole treatments to standard commercial tablets (%RB), the investigated treatments can be arranged, in descending order, as follows: metronidazole tablets containing CMC in drug: polymer ratio 1:1(treatment III), metronidazole tablets containing methyl cellulose in drug: polymer ratio 2:1 (treatment IV), metronidazole tablets containing Carbopol 934 in drug: polymer ratio 2:1 (treatment II), metronidazole capsules containing pectin in drug: polymer ratio 1:2 (treatment VI), and metronidazole capsules containing HPMC 15000 in drug: polymer ratio 2:3 (treatment V).

Though, with respect to the aforementioned parameters, treatment III which is metronidazole tablets containing CMC in drug: polymer ratio 1:1 was found to be the best studied treatment as it showed short t_{max}, medium C_{max}, medium MRT, good K_{ab}, and the best relative bioavailability.

372

REFERENCES

➢ **AAPS/FDA Workshop Committee. (1995).** Scale-up of oral extended-release dosage forms. Pharm. Tech., 19:46-54.

➢ **Abd El-Hameed-IM. (1996).** Studies on the Formulation, Bioavailability and Clinical Evaluation of Certain Angiotensen Converting Enzyme Inhibitors. PhD thesis, Cairo University. Egypt. Faculty of pharmacy.

➢ **Agyilirah-GA; Green-M; DuCret-R; Banker-GS. (1991).** Evaluation of the gastric retention properties of a cross-linked polymer coated tablet versus those of a non-disintegrating tablet. Int. J. Pharm., 75: 241-247.

➢ **Allroggen-H; Abbott-RJ;Bibby-K.(2000).** Acute visual loss following administration of metronidazole: a case report.Neuro-ophthalmol.23, 89-94.

➢ **Alvisi-V; Gasparetto-A; Dentale-A; Heras-H; felletti-spadazzi-A; D'apobrosi-A. (1996).** Bioavailability of a controlled release formulation of ursodeoxycholic acid in man. Drugs Exp. Clin. Res., 2229-33.

➢ **AMA-Department of Drugs. (1983).** AMA Drug Evaluations, 5th ed. American Medical Association, Chicago, IL.

➢ **Amaral-Moraes-ME; De-Pierossi-M; Moraes-MO; Bezerra-FF; Ferrira-Da-Silva-CM; Dias-HB; Muscara-MN; De-Nucci-G; Pedrazzoli-J. (1996).** Short-term sucralfate administration does not alter the absorption of metronidazole in healthy male volunteers.Int.J.Clin.Pharmacol.Ther., 34: 433-437.

➢ **Amon-I; Amon-K; Huller-H. (1980).** Int. J. Clin. Pharmacol., 26: 231.

➢ **Amon-I; Amon-K; Scharp-H. (1983).** Disposition kinetics of metronidazole in children.Eur.J.Clin.Pharmacol., 24,113-119.

➢ **Anon. (1976).** Metronidazole (Flagyle (R)) box warning. FDA Drug Bull.6:22.

➢ **Anon. (1995).** Drugs for parasitic infections. Med. Lett. Drugs. Ther., 37: 99-107.

➢ **Ansel-HC; Popvich-NC; Allen-LV. (1999).** Modified-Release Dosage Forms and Drug Delivery Systems,in: Pharmaceutical Dosage Forms And Drug Delivery Systems, 7th Ed.,Balado,D, (ed) Williams and Wilkins, Lea and Febiger Book, USA, pp 229-243.

➢ **Asrani-K. (1994).** Evaluation of bioadhesive properties of poly (acrylic acid) polymers and design of a novel floating bioadhesive drug delivery system. Doctoral thesis. St. John's University. Jamaica. N.Y.

➢ **Atyabi-F; Sharma-HL; Mohammad-HAH; Fell-JT. (1994).** A novel floating system using ion exchange resins, proc. Int. Symp. Control. Rele. Bioact. Mater., 21: 806-807.

➢ **Atyabi-F; Sharma-HL; Mohammad-HAH; Fell-JT. (1996a).** Controlled drug release from coated floating ion exchange resin beads. J. Control. Rele., 42: 25-28.

➢ **Atyabi-F; Sharma-HL; Mohammad-HAH; Fell-JT. (1996b).** In vivo evaluation of a novel gastric retentive formulation based on ion exchange resins. J. Control. Rele., 42: 105-113.

➢ **Axon-ATR. (1991).** Helicobacter pylori therapy: effect on peptic ulcer disease, J. Gastroenterol. Hepatol., 6: 131-137.

➢ **Babu-NBM; Khar-RK. (1990).** In vitro and in vivo studies of sustained-release floating dosage forms containing salbutamol sulfate, Pharmazie., 45: 268-270.

➢ **Baker-RW; Lonsdale-HK. (1974).** in "Controlled Release of Biologically Active Agents", Tanquaty, A.C and Locey, R.E.(ed.), Plenum Press, New York, pp.15-71.

➢ **Balaban-DH; Peura-DA. (1997).** Helicobacter pylori-associated peptic ulcer and gastritis, in: "Gastrointestinal infections, Diagnosis and Management", LaMont, J.T. (Ed.), Marcel Dekker, New York, pp. 29-69.

➢ **Barnes-AR;Sugden-JK: (1986).**Pharm.ActaHelv.,61,218.

➢ **Basly-JP;Duroux-JL;Bernard-M.(1996).**Gamma radiation induced effect on metronidazole. Int. J. Pharm., 139: 219-221.

➢ **Baumgartner-S; Krist-J; Vrecer-F; Vodopivec-P; Zorko-B. (2000).** Optimization of floating matrix tablets and evaluation of their gastric residence time.Int. J. Pharm., 15; 195(1-2):125-35.

➢ **Bechgaard-H; Christensen-FN; Davis-SS; Hardy-JG; Taylor-MJ; Whalley-DR; Wilson-CG. (1985).** Gastrointestinal transit of pellet systems in ileostomy subjects and the effect of density. J. Pharm. Pharmacol., 37: 718-721.

➢ **Bechgaard-H; Ladefoged-K. (1978).** Distribution of pellets in the gastrointestinal tract. The influence on transit time exerted by the density or diameter of pellets. J. Pharm. Pharmacol., 30: 690-692.

➢ **Bennett-CE; hardy-JG; Wilson-CG. (1984).** The influence of posture on the gastric emptying of antacid. Int. J. pharm., 21: 18-24.

➢ **Bennett-WM; Aronoff-GR; Golper-TA. (1994).** Drug prescribing in renal failure:Dosing Guidelines for adults ,3 rd ed.,American College of Physocians,Philadelphia,PA.

➢ **Bergan-T; Arnold-E. (1980).** Int. J. Clin. Pharmacol., 26: 231.

➢ **Bielecka-Grzela-S; Klimowicz-A. (2003).** Application of cutaneous microdialysis to evaluate metronidazole and its main metabolite concentrations in the skin after a single oral dose. J. Clin. Pharm. Ther., 28(6):465-9.

➢ **Bingley-PJ; Harding-GM. (1987):** Clostridium difficile colitis following treatment with metronidazole and vancomycin. Postgrad Med. J., 63: 993-994.

➢ **Blaser-MJ. (1992).** Hypotheses on the pathogenesis and natural history of helicobacter pylori-induced inflammation. Gastroenterology, 102: 720-727.

➢ **Blum-AL. (1994).** Helicobacter pylori and peptic ulcer disease. Scand.J. Gastroenterol., 31 (Suppl.214):24-27.

➢ **Blum-AL. (1996).** Helicobacter pylori and peptic ulcer disease, Scand, J. Gastroenterol., 31 (Suppl). 21: 424-27.

➢ **Bogentoft-C. (1982).** Oral controlled-release dosage forms in perspective. Pharm. Int., 3: 366-369.

➢ **Bogner-RH. (1997).** Bioavailability and bioequivalence of extended-release oral dosage forms. US Pharmacist,22 (Suppl): 3-12.

➢ **Boren-T; Falk-P; Roth-KA; et al., (1993).** Attachment of Helicobacter pylori to human gastric epithelium mediated by blood group antigens. Science., 262: 1892-1895.

➢ **Boyce-EG; Cookoson-ET; Bond-WS. (1990).**Persistent metronidazole-induced peripheral neuropathy.DICP-Ann Pharmacother.,24: 19-21.

➢ **Braga-PC. (1991).** Antibiotic penetrability into bronchial mucus: pharmacokinetics and clinical considerations.Curr.Ther.Res.,49: 300-327.

➢ **Brahma-NS; Kwon-HK.(2000).** Floating drug delivery systems: approaches to oral controlled drug delivery via gastric retention. J. Cont. Rele., 63: 235-259.

➢ **Brandt-LJ; Bernstein-LH; Boley-SJ; Frank-MS. (1982)**.Gastroenterology.83: 383.

➢ **British Pharmacopea. (1993).** The Pharmaceutical Press, London, p 753.

➢ **Brogden-RN; Heel-RC; Speight-TM; Avery-GS. (1978).** Drugs.16: 387-417.

➢ **Bruce-TA. (1971).** Dark urine related to metronidazole therapy. JAMA. 218-1832.

➢ **Bulgarelli-E; Forni-F; Bernabei-MT.(2000)**.Effect of matrix composition and process conditions on casein-gelatin beads floating properties.Int. J. Pharm. 198 (2): 157-65.

➢ **Burton-S; Washington-N; Steele-RJC. (1995).** "Intragastric Distribution of Ion-Exchange Resins: A Drug Delivery System for the Topical Treatment of the Gastric Mucosa. J. pharm. Pahrmacol. 47: 901-906.

➢ **Caldwell-LJ; Gardner-CR; Cargil-RC. (1988a).** Drug delivery device which can be retained in the stomach for controlled period of time. US Patent 4: 735-804.

➢ **Caldwell-LJ; Gardner-CR; Cargil-RC; Higuchi-T. (1988b).** Drug delivery device which can be retained in the stomach for controlled period of time. US Patent 4: 758-836.

➢ **Cano-SB; Golgiewicz-FL. (1986).** Storage requirements for metronidazole injection. Am. J. Hosp. Pharm. 43: 2983-2985.

➢ **Cargill-R; Caldwell-LJ; Engle-K; Fix-JA; Porter-PA; Gardner-CR. (1988)**.Controlled gastric emptying. 1. Effect of physical properties on gastric residence times of non-disintegrating geometric shapes in beagle dogs. Pharm. Res. 5: 533-536.

➢ **Chang-HS; Park-H; Kelly-P; Robinson-JR. (1985).** Bioadhesive Polymer as Platform for Oral Controlled Drug Delivery. II. Synthesis and Evaluation of Some Swelling Water Insoluble Bioadhesive Polymers. J. Pharm. Sci. 74: 399-405.

➢ **Chen-CL; Hao-WH. (1998).**in-Vitro performance of floating sustained-release Capsules of Verapamil. Drug Dev. Ind. Pharm. 24: 1067-1072.

➢ **Chien-Y.E. (1983).** Drug Dev. Ind. Pharm 9, 1291.

➢ **Chien-YW. (1992).** Novel Drug Delivery Systems, Marcel Dekker, Inc. , New York, , p.162.

➢ **Chitnis-VS; Malshe-VS; Lalla-JK. (1991).** Bioadhesive polymers-synthesis, evaluation and application in controlled release tablets. Drug Dev. Ind. Pharm. 17: 879-892.

➢ **Choi-BY; Park-HJ; Hwang-Sj; Park-JB. (2002).** Preparation of alginate beads for floating drug delivery system: effects of CO_2 gas-forming agents. Int. J. Pharm. 4; 239(1-2): 81-91.

➢ **Chowcat-NL; Wyllie-JH. (1976).** Intravenous metronidazole in amoebic enterocolitis(letter). Lancet. 2 : 1143.

➢ **Chueh- HR; Zia-H; Rhodes-CT. (1995).** Optimization of sotalol floating and bioadhesive extended release tablet formulations. Drug Dev. Ind. Pharm.21: 1725-1747.

➢ **Chungi-VS; Dittert –LW; Smith –RB. (1979).** "Gastrointestinal Sites of furosemide Absorption in rates," Int. J. Pharm. 4, 27-38.

➢ **Cooreman-MP; Krausgrill-P; Hengels-KJ. (1993).** Local gastric and serum amoxicillin concentrations after different oral application forms, Antimicrob. Agents Chemother. 37: 1506-1509.

➢ **Coupe-AJ; Davis-SS; Wilding-IR. (1991).** Variation in gastriontestinal transit of pharmaceutical dosage forms in healthy subjects. Pharm. Res. 8: 360-364.

➢ **Cremer-K. (1997)."Drug** Delivery: Gastro-Remaining Dosage Forms," Pharm. J. 259: 108.

➢ **Crevoisier-C; Hoevels-B; Zueher-G; Da-Prada-M. (1987).** Bioavailability of dopa after madopar HBS administration in healthy volunteers. Eur. Neurol. 27: 365-465.

➢ **Cummingham-FE; Kraus-DM; Brubaker-L. (1994).** Pharmacokinetics of intravaginal metronidazole gel. J. Clin. Pharmacol. 34: 1060-1065.

➢ **Cummingham-FE; Kraus-DM; Brubaker-L. (1994).** Pharmacokinetics of intravaginal metronidazole gel. J. Clin. Pharmacol. 34: 1060-1065.

➢ **Current Good Manufacturing Practice. (1980).** 21 CFR 211.Food and Drugs part 211.

➢ **Dahi-MV; Katz-HI; Kruger-GG et al. (1998).**Topical metronidazole maintains remissions of rosacea. Arch. Dermatol. 134 : 676-683.

➢ **Dalia-MMG. (2002).** Biopharmaceutical Studies on Certain Antihypertensive Drugs in Controlled Release Delivery Systems. PhD thesis, Cairo University. Egypt. Faculty of pharmacy.

➢ **Das-T; Banerjee-S; Samuel-G; Sarma-HD; Korde-A; Venkatesh-M; Pillai-MR. (2003).** 99mTc-labeling studies of a modified metronidazole and its biodistrbution in tumor bearing animal models. Nucl Med Biol. 30 (2): 127-34.

➤ **David-FL; Da-Silva-CMF; Mendes-FD; Perraz-JGP; Muscara-MN; Moreno-HJr; De-Nucci-G; Pedrazzoli-R. (1998).** Acid suppression by omeprazole does not affect orally administered metronidazole bioavailability and metabolism in healthy male volunteers. Aliment. Pharmacol. Ther. 12: 349-354.

➤ **Davis-SS; Hardy-JG; Taylor-MJ; Whalley-DR; Wilson-CG. (1984).** Effect of food on the gastrointestinal transit of pellets and an osmotic device (Osmet). Int. J. Pharm. 21: 331-340.

➤ **Davis-SS; Stockwell-AF; Taylor-MJ; Hardy-JG; Whalley-DR; Wilson-CG; Bechgaard-H; Christensen-FN.(1986).** The effect of density on the gastric emptying of single and multiple-unit dosage forms. Pharm. Res.3: 208-213.

➤ **DeCrosta-MT; Jain-NB; Rudnic-EM. (1987).** U.S. Patent 4: 666-705.

➤ **Degtiareva-II; Bogdanov-A; Khatib-Z; Kharchenko-NV; Lodianaia-EV; Palladina-OL; Opanasiuk-ND. (1994).** The use of 3rd generation antacid preparations for the treatment of patients with nonulcerous dyspepsia and peptic ulcer complicated by reflux esophagitis. Likars' Ka Sprava 5-6, 119-122.

➤ **Dennis-A; Timmins-P; Lee-K. (1992).** Buoyant controlled release powder formulation.US Patent 5, 169, 638.

➤ **Desai-S. (1984).** A novel floating controlled release drug delivery system based on a dried gel matrix. M.S. thesis. St. John's University, Jamaica. NY.

➤ **Desai-S; Bolton-S. (1989).**Floating sustained release therapeutic compositions, U.S. Patent, 4.814, 179 :

➤ **Desai-S; Bolton-S. (1993).** Floating controlled-release drug delivery systems: in vitro-in vivo evaluation. pharm. Res. 10: 1321-1325.

➢ **Deshpande-AA; Shab-NH; Rhodes-CT; Malick-AW. (1997).** Development of a novel controlled release systemfor gastric retention. Pharm. Res. 14: 815-819.

➢ **Deshpande-AA;Rhodes-CT; Shah-NH; Malick-AW. (1996).** controlled- release drug delivery systems for prolonged gastric residence: an overview. Drug Dev. Ind. Pharm. 22(6): 531-539.

➢ **Diao-Y; Tu-XD. (1991).** Development and pharmacokinetic study of miocamycin sustained release tablets remaining floating in the stomach, Yao Hsuch Hsuch Pao .26: 695-700.

➢ **Dreger-IM; Gleason-PP; Chowdhry-TK. (1998).** Intermittent-dose metronidazole-induced peripheral neuropathy (letter). Ann. Pharmaco.Ther. 32: 267-268.

➢ **Drewe-J; Beglinger-C; Kissel-T. (1992).** "The Absorption Site of Cyclo- sporin in the Human GIT,"Br. Clin. Pharmacol. 33: 39-43.

➢ **Dykes-P; Hill-S; Marks-R. (1997).** Pharmacokinetic of topically applied metronidazole in two different formulations. Skin. Pharmacol. 10: 28-33.

➢ **Dzink-J; Bartlett-JG. (1980).** In vitro susceptibility of clostridium difficile isolates from patients with antibiotic-associated diarrhea or colitis. Antimicrob .Agents.Chemother. 17: 695-698.

➢ **Edwards-LJ. (1950).**Trans.Faraday Soc.,47: 723

➢ **El-Gibaly-I. (2002).** Development and in-vitro evaluation of novel floating chitosan microcapsules for oral use: comparison with non-floating chitosan microspheres. Int. J. Pharm. 249(1-2):7-21.

➢ **El-Kamel-AH; Sokar-MS; AlGamal-SS; Naggar-VF. (2001).** Preparation and evaluation of ketoprofin floating oral delivery system. Int. J. Pharm. 220(1-2):13-21.

➤ **Emi-W; Held-K. (1987).**The hydordynamically balanced system: a novel principle of controlled drug release. Eur. Neurol. 27 21-27.

➤ **Eradiri-O; Jamali-F; Thomson-ABR. (1988).** Interaction of metronidazole with Phenobarbital, cimitedine, prednisone, and sulfasalazine in Crohn's disease.Biopharm.Drug.Dispos.9: 219-227.

➤ **Erni-w; Held-K. (1987).** The Hydrodynamically balanced system: a novel principle of controlled drug release. Eur. Neurol. 27: 218-278.

➤ **Fabregas-JL; Claramunt-J; Cucala-J; Pous-R; Siles-A. (1994).** In-vitro testing of an antacid formulation with prolonged gastric residence time (Almagate Flot-Coat). Drug Dev. Ind. Pharm. 20: 1199-1212.

➤ **FDA guidelines (1987).** Guidelines for submitting documentation for the stability of Humans, Drugs and Biologics.FDA, Center for Drugs and Biologics. Office of drug research review. In Remington's Pharmaceutical Sciences, 20 th ed., p 986.

➤ **Fell-JT. (1996).** Targeting of drugs and delivery system to specific sites in the gastrointestinal tract. J. Anat. 189: 517-519.

➤ **Fix-JA; Cargill-R; Engle-K. (1993).** Controlled gastric emptying. III. Gastric residence time of a nondisintegrating geometric shape in human volunteers, Pharm. Res. 10: 1087-1089.

➤ **Ford-WD; Mackellar-A; Richardson-CJ. (1980).** Pre and postoperative rectal metronidazole for the prevention of wound infection in childhood appendicitis.J.Pediatr.Surg.15:160-163.

➤ **Franz-MR; Oth-MP. (1993).** Sustained release. Bilayer buoyant dosage form, US Patent 5, 232, 704.

➤ **Fredricsson-B; Hagstrom-B; Nord-CE. (1987):** Systemic concentrations of metronidazole and its main metabolites after intravenous, oral and vaginal administration. Gynecol.Obstet. Invest., 24: 200-207.

➢ **Freeman-CD; Klutman-NE; Lamp-KC. (1997).** Metronidazole: a therapeutic review and update.Drugs.54: 679-708.

➢ **Fujimori-J; Machida-Y; Nagai-T. (1994).** Preparation of magnetically responsive tablet and confirmation of its gastric residence in beagle dogs. STP Pharm. Sci., 4: 425-430.

➢ **Fujimori-J; Machida-Y; Tanaka-S; Nagai-T. (1995).** Effect of magnetically controlled gastric residence of sustained release tablets on bioavailability of acetaminophen. Int. J. Pharm. 119: 47-55.

➢ **Fung-HL. (1996).**in modern Pharmaceutics,3rd ed., Banker-GS; Rhodes-CT, ed., Marcel Dekker, New York, PP 209-237 (1996). Hunter-WJ; Hunter-JS, Statistics for experiments; An introduction to design, Data analysis, and Model Building, New york, John Wiley (1978).

➢ **Galcone-M; Nizzola-L; Cacioli-D; Mosie-G. (1981).** In-vitro Demonstration of Delivery Mechanism from Sustained release pellets. Curr. Ther. Res. 29: 217-234.

➢ **Galmier-MJ; Frasey-AM; Bastide-M; Beyssac-E; Petit-J; Aiache-JM; Lartigue-Mattei-C. (1998).** Simple and sensitive method for determination of metronidazole in human serum by high-performance liquid chromatography.J.Chromatogr.b.Biomed.Appl.720: 239-243.

➢ **Garret-ER. (1956). J.** Am. Pharm. Ass. Sci. Ed., 45: 195.

➢ **Gascon-AR; Gutierrez-Aragon-G; Hernandez-RM; Errasti-J; Pedraz-JL. (2003).**Pharmacokinetics and tissue penetration of pefloxacin plus metronidazole after administration as surgical prophylaxis in colorectal surgery. Int. J. Clin. Pharmacol. Ther. 41(6): 267-74.

➤ **Gattavecchia-E; Tonelli-D; Breccia-A. (1981).** J. Chromatogr. 224: 465.

➤ **Gehvrke-SH; Lee-PI. (1990).** In 'Specialized Drug Delivery Systems',Marcel Dekker. Inc.New York, 1st ED.,p 255.

➤ **Gerogiannis-VS; Rekkas-DM; Dallas-PP; Choulis-NH. (1994).**Effect of several factors on the floating and swelling characteristics of tablets. Use of experimental design techniques. Proc. Int. Symp. Control. Rele. Bioact. Mater.21: 808-809.

➤ **Gerogiannis-VS; Rekkas-DN; Dallas-PP; Choulis-NH. (1993).**Drug Development and Industerial Pharmacy. 19(9): 1061.

➤ **Giron-JA; Ozoktay-S. (1984).** Bacteroides fragilis pelvic abscess: resolution with metronidazole therapy alone. South .Med.J.77: 232-234.

➤ **Gjerloff-C; Arnold-E. (1982).** Pharmacokinetics of intravenous metronidazole in man.Acta.Pharmacol.Toxicol.51: 132-135.

➤ **Gold-BD-M; Huesca-PM; Sheman, et al., (1993).** Helicobacter mustelae and Helicobacter pylori bind to common lipid receptors in-vitro. infect. Immun. 61: 2632-2638.

➤ **Graham-DY. (1996).** Non-steroidal anti-inflammatory drugs, Helicobacter pylori and ulcers: where we stand. Am. J. Gastroenterol. 91:2080-2086.

➤ **Groning-R; Heun-G. (1984).** Oral dosage forms with controlled gastrointestinal transit. Drug Dev. Ind. Pharm. 10: 527-539.

➤ **Gupta-PK; Robinson-JR. (1988).** Gastric emptying of liquids in the fasted dog. Int. J. Pharm. 43: 45- 52.

➤ **Gupta-SK. (1987).**Stability studies of ampicillin floating tablets (Ampiflot) and buffered Ampiflot. MS.Thesis,St.John's University.

➢ **Gustafson-JII; Weissamn-I; Weinfeld-RE; Holazo-AA; Khoo-KC; Kaplan-SA. (1981).** Clinical bioavailability evaluation of a controlled release formulation of diazepam. J. pharmacokinetic. Bioharm. 9: 676-691.

➢ **Gu-TH; Chen-SX; Zhu-JB; Song-DJ; Guo-JZ; Hou-HM. (1992).** Pharmacokinetics and pharmacodynamics of dilitiazem floating tablets. Chung Kuo Yao Li Hsueh Pao.13: 527-534.

➢ **Haller-I. (1982).** In--vitro activity of the two principal oxidative metabolites of metronidazole against bacteroides fragilis and related species. Antimicrob. Agents.Chemother. 22: 165-166.

➢ **Hanauer-SB. (1996).**Inflammatory bowel disease. Nengl. J. Med. 344: 841-848.

➢ **Harder-S; Fuhr-U; Bergmann-D. (1990).**"Ciprofloxacin Absorption in "Different Regions of the Human GIT. Investigations with the hf Capsule, "Br. J. Clin. Pharmacol. 30: 35-39.

➢ **Haring-N; Salama-Z; Jaeger-H. (1988).** Triple quadropole mass spectrometric determination of bromoeriptine in human plasma with negative ion chemical ionization. Arzneim. Forsch. 38: 1529-1532.

➢ **Hashim-H; Li Wan Po-A. (1987).** Improving the release characteristic of water-soluble drugs form hydrophilic sustained release matrices by in situ gas-generation, Int. J. pharm. 35: 201-209.

➢ **Heatley-RV. (1992).** The treatment of Helicobacter pylori infection. Aliment. Pharmacol. Ther. 6: 291-303.

➢ **Heisterberg-L; Branebjerg-PE. (1983).** Blood and milk concentrations of metronidazole in mothers and infants.J.Perinat.Med. 11:114-120.

➢ **Hestin-D;Hanesse-B;Frimat-L.(1994).**Metronidazole-associated hepatotoxicity in a hemodialyzed patient (letter).Nephron.68,286.

➤ **Higuchi-T. (1963).** Mechanism of sustained action medication. J. Pharm. Sci. 52: 1145-1149.

➤ **Higuchi-T; Hovigna-A; Busse-LW. (1950).** J. Am. Pharm. Ass., Sci.Ed., 39, 405.

➤ **Hilton-AK; Deasy-PB. (1992).** In-vitro and In-vivo evaluation of an oral sustained-release floating dosage form of amoxicillin trihydrate. Int. J. Pharm. 86: 79-88.

➤ **Hinder-R; Kelly-K. (1977).**Canine gastric emptying of solids and liquids. Am. J. Physiol. 233: E 335-E340.

➤ **Hixson-AW; Crowell-JH. (1977).** in 'Pharmaceutics of solids and solid dosage forms',Wiley,New York.

➤ **Hoffman-JS; Katz-LM; Cave-DR. (1999).** Efficacy of a 1-week regimen of ranitidine bismuth citrate in combination with metronidazole and clarithromycin for Helicobacter pylori eradication.Aliment.Pharmacol.Ther.13: 503-506.

➤ **Hoffmann-C; Focke-N; Franke-G; Zschiesche-M; Siegmund-W. (1995).** Comparative bioavilability of metronidazole formulations (Vagimid) after oral and vaginal administration. Int. J. Clin. Pharmacol.Ther. 33. 232-239.

➤ **Horowitz-M; Maddox-A; Bochner-M; Wishart-J; Krevsky-B; Collins-P; Shearman-D. (1989).** Relationship between gastric emptying of solid and caloric liquid meals and alcohol absorption. Am. J. Physiol. 257: G291-G298.

➤ **Houghton-GW; Dennis-MJ; Gabriel-R. (1985).** Pharmacokinetics of metronidazole in patients with varying degrees of renal failure.Br.J.Clin.pharmacol.19: 203-209.

➤ **Houghton-GW; Thome-PS; Smith-J. (1979).**Comparison of the pharmacokinetics of metronidazolein healthy female volunteers following either a single oral or intravenous dose.Br.J.Clin.Pharmacol.8: 337-341.

➤ **Hunt-J; Stubbs-D. (1975).** The volume and energy content of meal as determinants of gastric-emptying. J. Physiol.245: 209-225.

➤ **Hwang-SJ; Park-H; Park-K. (1998).**Gastric retentive drug delivery systems. Crit. Rev. Ther. Drug carrier Syst. 15: 243-284.

➤ **Iannucccelli-V; Coppi-G; Leo-E; Fontana-F; Bernabei-MT. (2000).** PVP solid dispersions for the controlled release of furosemide from a floating multiple-unit system. Drug Dev. Ind. Pharm. 26(6):595-603.

➤ **Iannuccelli-V; Coppi-G; Bernabei-MT; Cameroni-R. (1998b).** Air compartment multiple-unit system for prolonged gastric residence. Part I. Formulation study. Int. J. Pharm. 174: 47-54.

➤ **Iannuccelli-V; Coppi-G; Sansone-R; Ferolla-G. (1998a).** Air compartment multiple-unit system for prolonged gastric residence. Part II. In vivo evaluation. Int. J. Pharm. 174: 55-62.

➤ **Ichikawa-M; Watanabe-S; Miyake-Y. (1989).** Granule remaining in stomach, US Patent 4, 844, 905.

➤ **Ichikawa-M;Watanabe-S; Miyake-Y. (1991).** A new multiple-unit oral floating dosage system. I: In-vitro evaluation of floating and sustained-release characteristics .J. Pharm. Sci. 80: 1062- 1066.

➤ **Ingani-HM; Timmemans-J; Moes-AJ. (1987).** Conception and in-vivo investigation of peroral sustained release floating dosage forms with enhanced gastrointestinal transit. Int. J. pharm. 35: 157-164.

➤ **Inouye-H; Yamamoto-I; Tanida-N; et al., (1989).** Helicobacter pylori in Japan: bacteriological fracture and prevalence in healthy subjects and patients with gastrodoudenal disorders. Gastroenterol. Jpn.24: 494-504.

➢ **Ioannides-LB; Somogyi-A; Spicer-J, et al. (1981).** Rectal administration of metronidazole provides therapeutic plasma levels in post-operative patients. N. Engl. J. Med. 305: 1569-1570.

➢ **Itoh-T; Higuchi-T; Gardner-CR; Caldwell-L. (1986).** Effect of particle size and food on gastric residence time of non-disintegrating solids in beagle dogs. J. Pharm. Pharmacol. 38: 801-806.

➢ **Jacoberger-B; Ubeaud-G; Rohr-S; Pain-L; Koffel-JC. (2000).** Tissue diffusion of metronidazole according to two routes of administration: Intravenous and rectal.J.Pharm.Clin.19/3: 219-222.

➢ **Jayanthi-G; jayaswal-SB; Srivastava-AK. (1995).** Formulation and Evaluation of terfenadine microballoons for oral controlled release. Pharmazie. 50: 769-770.

➢ **Jensen-JC; Gugler-R. (1983).**Single and multiple dose metronidazole kinetics. Clin. Pharmacol. Ther. 34: 481-487.

➢ **Jens-T-Carstensen; Rhodes-CT. (2000).** In Drug Stability Principles and Practices. 3rd Eds, Volume 107.p 2:319-329.

➢ **Jessa-MJ; Barrett-DA; Shaw-PN; Spiller-RC. (1996).** Rapid and selective high-performance liquid chromatographic method for the determination of metronidazole and its active metabolite in human plasma, saliva, and gastric juice.J.Chromatogr.B.Biomed.Appl.677: 374-379.

➢ **Joseph-NJ; Lakshmi-S; Jayakrishnan-A. (2002).** A floating-type oral dosage form for piroxicam based on hollow polycarbonate microspheres: in vitro and in vivo evaluation in rabbits. J. Control. Rele. 79(1-3):71-9.

➢ **Kaniwa-N; Aoyagi-N; Ogata-H; Ejima-A. (1988).** Gastric Emptying of Enteric Coated Drug Preparations. II. Effect of size and Density of

Enteric Coated Drug Preparations and Food on the Gastric emptying rates in humans. J. Pharm. Dyn. 565-570.

➢ **Katayama-H; Nishinura-T; Ochi-S; Tsuruta-Y; Yamazaki-Y. (1999).** Sustained release liquid preparation using sodium alginate for eradication of helicobacter pylori. Biol. Pharm. Bull. 22 55-60.

➢ **Katz-M. (1976).**Parasitic infections.J.Pediatr.87:165.

➢ **Kawashima-Y; Niwa-T; Takeuchi-H; Hino-T; Itoh-Y. (1991).** Preparation of Multiunit Hollow Microsoheres (Microballoons) with Acrylic Resin Containing Tranilast and Their Drug release characteristics (in-Vitro) and Floating Behavior (in-vitro) . J. Controll. Rele. 16: 279-290.

➢ **Kawashima-Y; Niwa-T; Takeuchi-H; Hino-T; Itoh-Y. (1992).** "Hollow Microspheres for Use as a Floating Controlled Drug Delivery System in the Stomach". J. Pharm. Sci. 81, 135-140.

➢ **Kawashima-Y; Niwa-T; Takeuchi-H; Hino-T; Itoh-Y. (1993).** Role of the solvent –diffusion –rate modifier in a new emulsion solvent diffusion method for preparation of ketoprofen microspheres. Microencaps.10: 329-340.

➢ **Kaye-CM; Sankey-MG; Thomas-LA. (1980).** A rapid and specific semi-micro method involving high-pressure liquid chromatography for the assay of metronidazole in plasma, saliva, serum, urine and whole blood.Br.J.Clin.Pharmacol.9: 528-529.

➢ **Kedzierewiez-F; Thouvenot-P; LemutJ; Benenne-A; Hoffman-M; Maineent-P. (1999).** Evaluation of peroral silicone dosage forms in humans by gamma-scintigraphy. J. Control. Rele. 58: 195-205.

➢ **Kelly-KA. (1981).** Motility of the stomach and gastroduodenal junction, in Physiology of the Gastrointestinal Tract, L.R. Johnson, ed., Raven Press, New York, , pp. 393-410.

➢ Kendall-AT; Stark-E; Sugden-JK. (1989). Int.J.Pharm.57: 217.

➢ Khattar-D; Ahuja-A; Khar-RK. (1990). Hydrodynamically balanced systems as sustained release dosage forms of propranolol hydrochloride. Pharmazie. 45: 356-358.

➢ Kim-CK; Lee-EJ. (1992).Int. J. Pharm.79: 11.

➢ Korsmeyer-RW; Gurny-R; Deoelker-E; Buri-P; Pappas-NA. (1983). Mechanisms of potassium chloride form compressed, hydrophilic, polymeric matrices: effect of entrapped air. J. pharm. Sci. 72: 1189-1191.

➢ Kortelainen-P; Huttunen-R; Keireluoma-MI. (1982). Single dose intrarectal metronidazole prophylaxis against wound infection after appendectomy.Am.J.Surg.143: 244-245.

➢ Kosky-KT. (1969). J. Pharm.Sci.58: 560.

➢ Kowlek-WF; Bookwater-CN. (1971). Food Technol. 25: 1025.

➢ Krishnaiah-YS; Veer Raju-P; Dinesh Kumar-B; Jaryaram-B; Rama-B; Raju-V; Bhaskar-P. (2003). Pharmacokinetic evaluation of guar-based colon-targeted oral drug delivery systems of metronidazole in healthy volunteers. Eur. J. Drug Metab. Pharmacokinetic .28 (4): 287-94.

➢ Kumaresh-SS; Anandro-RK; Tejraj-MA. (2001). Development of hollow microspheres as floating controlled-release systems for cardiovascular drugs: preparation and release characteristics. Drug Dev. Ind. Pharm. 27: 507-515.

➢ Lanbeck-K; Lindstrom-B. (1979). J. Chromatogr. 162: 117.

➢ Lashman-L; Cooper-J. (1959). J. Am. Pharm. Ass. 48: 226.

> **Lau-AH; Emmons-K; Seligsohon-R.(1991).** Pharmacokinetics of intravenous metronidazole at different dosages in healthy subjects. Int. J. Clin. Pharmacol.Ther.Toxicol. 29: 386-390.

> **Lee-CL. (1996).** The nature of helicobacter pylori, Scand. J. Gastroenterol. 31(Suppl 214): 5-8.

> **Lee-CL; Tu-TC; Wu-CH et al. (1998).** One-Week low-dose triple therapy is effective in treating Helicobacter pylori-infected patients with bleeding peptic ulcers.J.Formos.Med.Assoc.97: 733-737.

> **Lee-JH; Park TG; Lee-YB; Shin-SC; Choi-HK. (2001).**Effect of adding non-volatile oil as a core material for the floating microspheres prepared by emulsion solvent diffusion method. J. Microencapsul. 18(1):65-75.

> **Lee-JH; Park-TG; Choi-HK. (1999).** Development of oral drug delivery system using floating microspheres. J. Microencapsul. 16: 715-729.

> **Lenaerts-NM; Gurnny-R. (1990).** In: Bioadhesive systems. CRC Press. Boca Raton.EL.

> **Lenaerts-VM; Gurny-R. (1994).** In: Bioadhesive Drug Delivery Systems, CRC Press, Boca Raton, FL.

> **Libo-Y; Jamshid-E; Reza-F. (1999).** A new intragastric delivery system for the treatment of Helicobacter pylori associated gastric ulcer: in vitro evaluation. J. Control. Rel. 57: 215-222.

> **Lin-HC; Doty-J; Reedy-T; Meyer-J. (1990).** Inhibition of gastric emptying by sodium oleate depends on length of intestine exposed to nutrient, Am. J. Physiol. 259: G1031-G1036.

> **Lipka-E, Amidon-GL. (1999).** Setting bioequivalence requirement for drug development based on preclinical data: optimizing on drug delivery systems. J. Control. Rel. 62 : 41-49.

➤ **Li-S; Lin-S, Daggy-BP; Mirchandani-HL; Chien-YW. (2002).**
Effect of formulation variables on the floating properties of gastric
floating drug delivery system. Drug Dev. Ind. Pharm. 28(7): 783-93.

➤ **Li-S; Lin-S; Daggy-BP; Mirchandani-HL; Chien-YW. (2003).**
Effect of HPMC and Carpobol on the release and floating properties
of gastric floating drug delivery System using factorial design. Int. J.
Pharm. 253(1-2):13-22.

➤ **Li-S;Lin-S; Chein-YW; Daggy-BP; Mirchandani-HL.
(2001).**Statistical optimization of gastric floating system for oral
controlled delivery of calcium. AAPS. Pharm. Sci. Tech. 13:2(1):E1.

➤ **Li-SL; Tu-XD; Mao-FF. (1989).** Development and pharmacokinetic
study of metoprolol tartarate controlled-release tablet remaining
floating in the stomach, Yao Hsuch Hsuch Pao .24: 381-386.

➤ **Little-GB; Boylan-JC. (1981).** Flagyl reacts with
aluminium.Hosp.Pharm.16: 627.

➤ **Loft-S;Otton-SV;Lennard-MS;Tucker-GT;Poulsen HE. (1991).**
Characterization of metronidazole metabolism by human liver
microsomes. Biochem. Pharmacol. 41, 1127-1134.

➤ **Logan-RPH. (1994).** Helicobacter pylori and gastric cancer, lancet.
344: 1078-1079.

➤ **Longer-MA; Ching-HS; Robinson-JR. (1985).** Bioadhesive
polymers as platforms for oral controlled drug delivery III: oral
delivery of chlorothiazide using a bioadhesive polymer. J. pharm. Sci.
74: 406- 411.

➤ **Lordi-NG. (1986).** In 'The theory and Practice of Industrial
Pharmacy', Lea and Febiger, Philadelphia, 3rd, p 430.

➢ **Lowe-NJ; Henderson-T; Millikan-LE et al. (1989).** Topical metronidazole for severe and recalcitrant rosacea: a prospective open trial.Cutis.43, 283-286.

➢ **Machida-Y; lnouye-K; Tokumura-T. (1989).** "Preparation and Evaluation of Intragastric Buoyant Preparations" drug des del. 4, 155-161.

➢ **Madan-PL. (1985a).** Sustained-release drug delivery systems: part II, prefomulation considerations. Pharmaceutical Manufacturing. 2:41-45.

➢ **Madan-PL. (1985b).** Sustained-release drug delivery systems: part I, an overview. Pharmaceutical Manufacturing. 2:23-27.

➢ **Madan-PL. (1990).** Sustained release dosage forms. US Pharmacist. 15:39-50.

➢ **Mahfouz-NM; Aboul-Fadl-T; Diab-AK. (1998).** Metronidazole twin ester prodrugs: Synthesis, physicochemical properties, hydrolysis kinetics and antigiardial activity.Eur.J.Med.Chem.33/9: 975-683.

➢ **Mahfouz-NM; Hassan-MA. (2001).** Synthesis, chemical and enzymatic hydrolysis, and bioavilability evaluation in rabbits of metronidazole amino acid ester prodrugs with enhanced water solubility.J.Pharm.Pharmacol.53/6:841-848.

➢ **Majoaverian-P; Reyonolds-JC; Ouyang-A; Wirth-F; Kellner-PE; Vlasses-PH. (1991).** Mechanism of gastric emptying of a nondisintegrating radiotelemetry capsule in man. Pharm. Res. 8: 97-100.

➢ **Malcolm-SL; Allen-JG; Bird-H; Quinn-NP; Marion-MH; Marsden-CD; O'Leary-CG. (1987).** Single-dose pharmacokinetics of Madopar HBS in patients and effect of food and antacid on the absorption of Madopar HBS in volunteers. Eur. Neurol. 27: 285-355.

➤ **Mamajek-RC; Moyer-ES. (1980).** Drug-dispensing device and method, U.S. Patent, 4,207,890.

➤ **Marques-RA; Stafford-B; Flynn-N; Sadee-W. (1978).** J. Chroatogr. 146: 163.

➤ **Marshall-BJ; Barrett-LJ; Prakash-C., et al., (1990).** Urea protects Helicobacter (Camplylobacter) pylori from the bactericidal effect of acid. Gastroenter. 99: 697-702.

➤ **Marshall-BJ; Warren-JR. (1984).** Unidentified curved bacilli in the stomach of patients with gastritis and peptic ulceration Lancet. 1311-1315.

➤ **Martin-A; Bustamante-P; Chun-AHC. (1993).** In 'Physical Pharmacy, Physical Chemical Principle in the Pharmaceutical Science', 4th Ed., Ch 9, Lea and Febiger, Philadelphia, London.

➤ **Martindale, The Extra Pharmacopeia,(1993),** 13th Ed., Reynolds-JEF(ed). Londone: The Pharmaceutical Press.

➤ **Matharu-RS; Sanghavi-NM. (1992).** "Novel Drug Delivery System for Captopril," Drug Dev. W. Pliarm. 18: 1567-1574.

➤ **Mathew-M; Cupta-VD; Bethea-C. (1993).** The development of oral liquid dosage forms of metronidazole. J.Clin.Pharm.Ther.18: 291-294.

➤ **Mathew-M; Cupta-VD; Bethea-C. (1994a).** Stability of metronidazole benzoate in suspensions. J.Clin. Pharm.Ther. 19: 31-34.

➤ **Mathew-M; Cupta-VD; Bethea-C. (1994b).** Stability of metronidazole in solutions and suspensions. J. Clin. Pharm.Ther. 19: 27-29.

➤ **Mathiowitz-E; Chickering-D; Jacob-J; Dibiase-M; Bernstein-H;Gunn-K; Sherman-M. (1994).** GI transit studies of hydrophobic protein microspheres, Proc. Int. Symp. Control. Rel. Bioact. Mater., 21: 27-28

➤ **Mazer-N; Abisch-E; Gfeller-JC; Laplanche-R;. Bauer feind-P; Cucala-M; Lukachich-M; Blum-A. (1988).** Intragastric behavior and absorption kinetics of a normal and "floating modified-release capsule of isradipine under fasted and fed conditions J. Pharm. Sci. 8: 647-657.

➤ **McEvoy-G, ed. (1995).** AHFS Drug Information 95.Bethesda, MD: American Society of Health-System Pharmacists.

➤ **Menon-A; Ritschel-WA; Sakr-A. (1994).** Development and evaluation of a monolithic floating dosage form for furosemide. J. Pharm. Sci. 83: 239-245.

➤ **Michael-E. (1990).** In Biopharmaceutics, The Science of Dosage Form Design, Michael, E., ed., Aulton, p. 174- 183.

➤ **Michaels-AS. (1974).** Drug delivery device with self actuated mechanism for retaining device in selected area, US Patent, 3, 786, 831.

➤ **Michaels-AS; Bashwa-JD; Zaffaroni-A. (1975).** Integrated device for administering beneficial drug at programmed rate, US, Patent, 3,901, 232.

➤ **Midha-KK; McGilverery-IJ; Cooper-JK. (1973).** J. Chromatogr. 87: 491.

➢ **Minami-H; McCallum-RW. (1984).**The physiology and pathophysiology of gastric emptying in humans. Gastoenter. 86: 1592-1610.

➢ **Miyazaki-S; Yamaguchi-H; Yokouchi-C; Takada-M; Hou-WM. (1988).** Sustained-release and intragastric-floating granules of indomethacin using chitosan in rabbits. Chem. Pharm. Bull. 36: 4033-4038.

➢ **Moes-AJ. (1993).** Gastroretentive dosage forms. Crit. Rev. Ther. Drug Carrier Syst. 10: 143-195.

➢ **Mojaverian-P; Ferguson-R; Vlasses-P; Rocci-M; Oren-A; Fix-J; Caldwell-L; Gardener-C. (1985).** Estimation of gastric residence time of the Heidelberg capsule in humans: effect on varying food composition, Gastroenter. 89: 392-397.

➢ **Mojaverian-P; Reynolds-JC; Ouyang-A; Wirth-F; Kellner-PE; Vlasses-PH. (1991).** Mechanism of gastric emptying of a non-disintegrating radioelementry capsule in man.Pharm.Res.8: 97-100.

➢ **Mojaverian-P; Vlasses-PH; Kellener-PE; Rocci-ML. (1988).** Effects of gender. Posture and age on gastric residence time of an indigestible solid: pharmaccutical considerations pharm. Res. 10: 639-644.

➢ **Mollica-JA; Ahuja-S; Cohen-J. (1978).** J. Pharm. Sci. 67: 443.

➢ **Moore-JG; Christian-PE; Brown-JA; Brophy-C; Datz-F Taylor-A; Alazraki-N. (1984).** Influence of meal weight and caloric content on gastric emptying of meals in man. Dig. Dis. Sci 29 513-519.

➢ **Moursy-NM; Afifi-NN; Gorab-DM, El-Saharty-Y. (2003).** Formulation and evaluation of susteained release floating capsules of nicardipine hydrochloride.Pharmazie. 58(1): 38-43.

➢ **Muller-lissner-SA; Blum-AL. (1981).** The effect of specific gravity and eating on-gastric emptying of slow-release capsules, New Engl. J. Med. 304 :1365-1366.

➢ **Murata-Y; Kofuji-K; Kawashima-S. (2003).** Preparation of floating alginate gel beads for drug delivery to the gastric mucosa.J. Biomater. Sci. Polym. Ed. 14(6):581-8.

➢ **Murata-Y; Sasaki-N; Miyamoto-E; Kawashima-S. (2000).** Use of floating alginate gel beads for stomach-specific drug delivery. Eur. J. Pharm. Biopharm. 50(2): 221-6.

➢ **Murthy-KS; Sellassie-IG. (1993).** J. Pharm. Sci. 82: 113.

➢ **Muscara-MN; Pedrazzoli-J; Miranda-EL; Ferraz-JG; Hofstatter-E; Leite-G; Magalhaes-AF; Leonardi-S; Denucci-S. (1995).** Plasma hydroxy-metronidazole/metronidazole ratio in patients with liver disease and in healthy volunteers. Br. J. Clin. Pharmacol.40: 477-480.

➢ **Nagar-H; Berger-SA; Hammar-B. (1989).** Penetration of clindamycin and metronidazole into the appendix and the peritoneal fluid in children. Eur.J.Clin.Pharmacol. 37:209-210.

➢ **NIH Consensus** Development Panel on Helicobacter pylori in Peptic Ulcer disease. **(1994).** Helicobacter pylori in Peptic Ulcer Disease.JAMA. 272: 65-69.

➢ **Nilsson-I; Ursing-B; Nilsson-P. (1981).** Antimicrob. Agents Chemother. 18: 754.

➢ **Norari-RE. (1971).** In Biopharmaceutics and Pharmacokinetics, Marcel Dekker, Inc, New York.

➢ **Nur-AO; Zhang-JS. (2000).** Captopril floating and/or bioadhesive tablets: design and release kinetics. Drug Dev. Ind. Pharm. 26(9): 965-9.

➤ O'Keefe-JP; Troc-KA; Thompson-KD. (1982). Activity of metronidazole and its hydroxy and acid metabolites against clinical isolates of anaerobic bacteria. Antimicrob.Agents.Chemother.22: 426-430.

➤ Okonkwo-PO; Eta-EI. (1988). Simultaneous determination of chloroquine and metronidazole in human biological fluid by high-pressure liquid chromatography.Life.Sci.42: 539-545.

➤ Oth-M; Franz-M; Timmermans-J; Moes-A. (1992). The bilayer floating capsule: a stomach-directed drug delivery sysem for misoprostol, Pharm, Res. 9: 298-302.

➤ Ozyazici-M; Turgut-EH; Taner-MS; Koseoglu-K; Ertan-G. (2003).In-vitro evaluation and vaginal absorption of metronidazole suppositories in rabbits. J. Drug Target. 111 (3):177-85.

➤ Palin-KJ; Whalley-DR; Wilson-CG; Davis-SS; Philips-AJ. (1982). Determination of gastric emptying in the rat: influence of oil structure and volume. Int. J. Pharm. 12: 315-322.

➤ Pargal-A; Toa-C; Bhopale-KK; Pradhan-KS; Masani-KB; Kaul-CL. (1993). Comparative pharmacokinetics and amoebicidal activity of metronidazole and satranidazole in the golden hamster, Mesocricetus auratus. J. Antimicrob.Chemother.32: 483-489.

➤ Park-H; Robinson-JR. (1985). Physico-chemical properties of water insoluble polymers important to mucin/epithelial adhesion. J. Control. Rel. 2: 45-57.

➤ Park-K; Robinson-JR. (1984).Biodhesive polymers as platforms for oral-controlled drug delivery: method to study bioadhesion. Int. J. Pharm. 19: 107-127.

➢ **Passmore-CM; McElnay-JC; Rainey-EA. (1988).** Metronidazole excretion in human milk and its effect on the suckling neonate. Br. J. Clin. Pharmacol. 26: 45-51.

➢ **Patel-VR; Amiji-MM. (1996).** "Preparation and Characterizations of Freezebiotic Delivery in the Stomach," Pharm. Res.13, 588-593.

➢ **Peng-DA Wang; Ming-Kung-YCH. (1993).** Degradation kinetics of metronidazole in solution. J. Pharm. Scie.82: 95-98.

➢ **Pharmaceutical Practice. (1990).** edited by Diane-M.Collett; Michael-E.Alton, p 45.

➢ **Phuapradit-W. (1989).** Influence of tablet buoyancy on the human oral absorption of sustained release acetaminophen tablets, Doctroal thesis, St, John's University, Jamaica. NY.

➢ **Phuapradit-W; Bolton-S. (1991).** The influence of tablet density on the human oral absorption of sustained release acetaminophen matrix tablets. Drug Dev. Ind. Pharm. 1097-1107.

➢ **Physician's Desk Refernce. (1993).**47th ed. Oradell-NJ: Medical Economics Company,

➢ **Pierleoni-EE. (1984).** Topical metronidazole therapy for infected decubitus ulcers. J. Am. Geriatr. Soc. 32: 775.

➢ **Pollak-PT. (1996).** A liquid chromatography assay for the study of serum and gastric juice metronidazole concentrations in the treatment of Helicobacter pylori.Ther. Drug.Monit.18: 678-687.

➢ **Ponchel-G; Touchard-E; wouessidiewe-D; Duchene-D; Peppas-NA. (1987).** Int. J. pharm. 38: 65.

➢ **Prantera-C; Berto-E; Scribano-ML. (1998).** Use of antibiotics in the treatment of active Crohn's disease:experience with metronidazole and ciprofloxacin. Ital. J. Gastroenterol. Hepatol. 30: 602-606.

➢ **Product Information. (1999).** Flagyl (R), metronidazole. Searle Labs, Chicago, IL, USA.

➢ **Product Information. (1999).** Noritate (R), metronidazole.Demik Laboratories,Collegeville,PA,USA.

➢ **Rajnarayana-K; Reddy-MS; Krishna-DR. (2003).** Diosmin pretreatment affects bioavailability of metronidazole. Eur. J. Clin. Pharmacol. 12: 803-7.

➢ **Rajnarayana-K; Reddy-MS; Vidyasagar-J; Krishna-DR. (2004).**Study on the influence of silymarin pretreatment on metabolism and disposition of metronidazole. Arzneimittelforschung. 54(2):109-13.

➢ **Ralph-ED. (1983).** Clinical pharmacokinetics of metronidazole.Clin.Pharm.8: 43-62.

➢ **Ralph-ED; Clarke-JT; Libke-RD. (1974).** Pharmacokinetics of metronidazole as determined by bioassay. Antimicrob.Agents.Chemother.6: 691-696.

REFERENCES

➢ **Regmi-BM; Liu-JP; Tu-XD. (1996).** Studies on ethmozine (EMZ) sustained release tablets, remaining-floating in stomach, Yao Hsuch Hsuch Pao 31: 54-58.

➢ **Remington's Pharmaceutical Sciences, (2000).**20th ed., Mack Publishing Co., Easton, Pennsylvania.

➢ **Rhodes-CT. (1984).** An over view of kinetics for the evaluation of the stability of pharmaceutical systems. Drug Dev. Ind. Pharm.10: 1163-1174.

➢ **Ritschel-WA. (1991).** Targeting in the gastrointestinal tract: new approaches, Methods find. Exp. Clin. Pharmacol. 13: 313-336.

➢ **Ritschel-WA; Menon-A; Saker-A. (1991).** Biopharmaceutic evaluation of furosemide as a potential candidate for a modified release peroral dosage form. Methods Find. Exp. Clin. Pharmacol. 13: 629-636.

➢ **Rogers-JD; Kwan-KC. (1979).** Pharmacokinetic requirements for controlled-release dosage forms. In: John Urquhart, ed. Controlled-release pharmaceuticals. Washington DC: Academy of Pharmaceutical Sciences, American Pharmaceutical Association. 95-119.

➢ **Rosenblatt-JE; Randall-SE. (1987).** Metronidazole. Mayo.Clin. Proc.62: 1013-1017.

➢ **Rouge-N; Allemann-E; Gex-Fabry-M; Balant-L; Cole-ET; Buri-P; Doclker-E. (1998b)** Comparative pharmacokinetie study of a floating multiple –unit capsule, a high-density multiple-unit capsule and an intermediate-release tablet containing 25 mg atenolol. Pharm. Acta Helv. 73: 81-87.

➢ **Rouge-N; Buri-P; Doelker-E. (1996).** Drug absorption sites in the gastrointestinal tract and dosage forms for site-specific delivery. Int. J. Pharm. 136: 117-139.

➢ **Rouge-N; Cole-ET; Doelker-E; Buri-P. (1998a).** Buoyancy and drug release patterns of floating minitablets containing piretanide and atenolol as model drugs, pharm Dev. Technol. 3 73-84.

➢ **Rubinstein-A; Friend-DR. (1994).** Specific delivery to the gastrointestinal tract. In: A.J. Domb (Ed.), Polymeric site-specific Pharmacotherapy. Wiley. Chichester, pp.282-283.

➢ **Rune-SJ. (1996).** History of Helicobacter pylori infection, Scnad. J. Gastroenterol. 31 (suppl. 214): 2-4.

➢ **Sah-H. (1997).** Microencapsulating techniques Using Ethyl Acetate as Dispersed solvent: effect of Its extraction rate on the characteristics of PLGA Microspheres. J. Control. Rel. 47: 233-245.

➢ **Sah-H; Smith-MS; Chern-Rt. (1996).**A Novel Method of Preparing PLGA Microspheres Utilizing Methyl 5 Ketone. Pharm. Res. 13: 360-367.

➢ **Salas-Herrera-IG; Lawson-M; Johnston-A; Turner-P; Gott-DM; Dennis-MJ. (1991).** Plasma metronidazole concentrations after single and repeated vaginal pessary administration.Br.J.Clin.Pharmacol.32: 651-623.

➢ **Sangekar-S; Vadino-WA; Chaudry-I; Parr-A; Beihn-R; Digenis-G. (1987).** Evaluation of the effect of food and specific gravity of tablets on gastric retention time, Int. J. Pharm. 35 : 187-191.

➢ **Sato-Y; Kawashima-Y; Takeuchi- H; Yamamoto-H. (2003).** In vivo evaluation of riboflavin-containing microballoons for floating controlled drug delivery system in healthy human volunteers. J. Control. Rel. 18; 93 (1):39-47.

➢ **Sato-Y; Kawashima-Y; Takeuchi- H; Yamamoto-H. (2004).** In vitro and in vivo evaluation of riboflavin-containing microballoons for a floating controlled drug delivery system in healthy humans. Int. J. Pharm. 4; 275 (1-2): 97-107.

➢ **Sattar-MA; Sankey-MG; Cawley-MI. (1982).**The penetration of metronidazole into synovial fluid. Postgrad. Med. J. 58: 20-24.

➢ **Schuster-O; Heartel-M; Hugemann-B. (1985).** "Untersuchung zur klinischen pharmacokinetic von Allopurinol," Arzneim. – Forsch. 35: 760-764.

➢ **Seta-Y; Higuchi-F; Otsuka-t; Kawahara-Y; Nishimura-K; Okada-R; Koike. (1988).** Int. J. pharm., 41, 255.

➢ **Shalaby-WSW; Blevins-E; Park-K. (1992 b)** Use of ultrasound imaging and fluoroscopic imaging to study gastric retention of enzyme-digestible hydrogels, Biomaterials. 13: 289-296.

➢ **Shalaby-WSW; Blevins-E; Park-K. (1992a)** In vitro and in-vivo studies of enzyme digestible hydrogels for oral drug delivery. J. Control. Rel. 19: 131-144.

➢ **Sheth-PR; Tossounian-JL. (1978).** Sustained release pharmaceutical capsules, U.S patent 4: 126, 672.

➢ **Sheth-PR; Tossounian-JL. (1979).** Novel sustained release Tablet formulation, US Patent 4: 167-558.

➢ **Sheth-PR; Tossounian-JL. (1984).**The Hydroynamically balanced system (HBS): a novel drug delivery system for oral use, Drug Dev. Ind. Pharm. 10: 313-339.

➢ **Shorgel-L; Yu-ABC. (1999).** in Applied Biopharmaceutics and Pharmacokinetics, 4^{rd}Ed., Ch.11, cheryl-LM, (eds), York Production Services, USA. pp. 281-323.

➢ **Siegal-J; Urbain-J; Adler-L; Charkes-N; Maurer-A; Krevsky-B; Knight-L; Fisher-R; Malmud-L. (1988).**Biphasic nature of gastric emptying. Gut. 29: 85-89.

➢ **Siegmund-W; Zschiesche-M; Franke-G; Wilke-A. (1992).** Bioavailability of metronidazole formulations (VagimidR). Pharmazie.47: 522-525.

➢ **Singh-BN. (1999).** Effects of food on clinical pharmacokinetics. Clin. Pharmacokinetic. 37:213-255.

➢ **Singh-BN; Kim-KH. (2000).** Floating Drug Delivery Systems: An Approach to Oral Controlled Drug Delivery via Gastric Retention. J. Control. Rel. 63: 235-259.

➢ **Slomiany-BL; Piotrowski-J; Samanta-A, et al., (1989).** Campylobacter pylori colonization factors shows specificity for lactosylceramide sulfate and GM3 ganglioside, Biochem, Int. 19: 929-936.

➢ **Smith-JA. (1980).** Neuropenia associated with metronidazole therapy.Can.Med.Assoc. J. 123:202.

➢ **Somogyi-AA; Kong-CB; Gurr-FW. (1984).** Metronidazole pharmacokinetics in patients with acute renal failure.J.Antimicrob.Chemother.13: 183-189.

➢ **Soppimath-KS; Kulkarni-AR; Aminabhavi-TM. (2001).** Development of hollow microsphres as floating controlled-release for cardiovascular drugs: preparation and release characteristics. Drug Dev. Ind. Pharm. 27(6):507-15.

➢ **Stambaugh-JE.Feo-LG; Manther-RW. (1968).** The isolation and identification of the urinary oxidative metabolites of metronidazole in man.J.Pharmacol.Exp.Ther.161: 373-381.

➢ **Stewart-JT; Maddex-FC; Warren-FW. (2000).** Stability of cefepime hydrochloride injection and metronidazole in poly vinyl chloride bags at 4 degree and 20 degree, -24 C degree. HOSP. Pharm. 35: 1057-1064.

➢ **Stockwell AF; Davis-SS; walker-SE. (1986).** In-vitro evaluation of alginate gel systems as sustained release drug delivery systems. J. Control. Rel. 3: 167-175.

➢ **Streubel-A; Siepmann-J; Bodmeier-R. (2002).**Floating microparticles based on low density foam powder. Int. J. Pharm. 25; 241(2):279-92.

➢ **Streubel-A; Siepmann-J; Bodmeier-R. (2003a).** Floating matrix tablets based on low density foam powder: effects of formulation and processing parameters on drug release. Eur. J. Pharm .Sci.18 (1): 37-45.

➢ **Streubel-A; Siepmann-J; Bodmeier-R. (2003b).** Multiple unit gastro retentive drug delivery systems: a new preparation method for low density microparticles. J .Microencapsul. 20(3): 329-47.

➢ **Struthers-BJ; Parr-RJ. (1985).** Clarifying the metronidazole hydrochloride-aluminum interaction. Am. J. Hosp. Pharm. 42: 2660.

➢ **Sujimori-J; Machida-Y; Nagai-T. (1994).**Preparation of magnetically responsive tablet and confirmation of its gastric residence in beagle dogs. STP Pharm. Sci. 4: 425-430.

➢ **Su-MH; Lee-PH; Ghanem-Ah; Higuchi-WI. (1991).** Clin. Pharm. J. 43.

➢ **Suwanee-PP; Tomomi-H; Tetsuya-A; Kazunori-K; Tamotsu-K. (1995).** Chem. Pharm. Bull. 43: 994.

➢ **Sweta-SHAH; Roula-Q; Vijay-P; Mansoor-A. (1999).** Evaluation of the factors influencing stomach-specific delivery of antibacterial agents for Helicobacter Pylori infection. J. Pharm. Pharmacol. 51: 667-672.

➢ **Tally-FP; Suttler-VL; Finegold-SM. (1975).** Treatment of anaerobic infections with metronidazole. Antimicrob. Agents. Chemother. 7: 672-675.

➢ **Tanaka-H; Matsumura-M; Veliky-IA. (1984).** Biotechnol.Bioeng. 26,53.

➢ **Tanner-WA; Ali-AE; Collins-PG. (1980).** Single dose intrarectal metronidazole as prophylaxis against wound infection following emergency appendectomy. Br. J. Surg. 67: 809-810.

➤ **Thanoo-BC; Thanoo- MC; Sunny-MC; Jayakrishnan-A. (1993).** Oral sustained release drug delivery systems using polycarbonate microspheres capable of floating on the gastric fluid. J. Pharm. Pharmacol. , 45: 21-24.

➤ **Timmeramans-J; Moes-AJ. (1994).** Factors controlling the buoyancy and gastric retention capabilities of floating matrix capsules: new data for reconsidering the controversy, J. Pharm. Sci. 83: 18-24.

➤ **Timmermans-J, Moes-AJ. (1990).** How well do floating dosage forms float. Int. J. Pharm. 62: 207-216.

➤ **Timmermans-J. (1990).** Comparative evaluation of the gastric transit of floating and non-floating matrix dosage forms. Bull, mem. Acad, R. Med, Belg. 145: 365-375.

➤ **Timmermans-J. (1991).** Floating hydrophilic matrix dosage forms for oral use: factors controlling their buoyancy and gastric residence capabilities, Ph.D. thesis, University of Brusseis.

➤ **Timmermans-J; Van Gansbeke-B; Moes-AJ. (1989).** Assessing by gamma scintegraphy the in vivo buoyancy of dosage forms having known size and floating force profiles as a function of time. Proc. 5th Int. Conf. Pharm. Technol. Vol.I, APGI, Paris. 42-51.

➤ **Todd-RS; Fryers-GR. (1979).** Cholestyramine compositions and method fro treating biliary gastritis. US Patent 4, 172, 129.

➤ **Triebling-AT; Korsten-MA; Dlugosz-JWQ, et al., (1991).** Severity of Helicobacter-induced gastric injury correlates with gastric Juice ammonia. Dig. Dis. Sci. 36: 1089-1096.

➤ **Tsai-TH; Chen- YF. (2003).** Pharmacokinetics of metronidazole in rat blood, brain, and bile studied by microdialysis coupled to microbore liquid chromatography. J. Chromatogr A. 14: 277- 82.

➢ **Tyburski-JG; Wilson-RF; Warsow-KM. (1998).** A trial of ciprofloxacin and metronidazole vs gentamicin and metronidazole for penetrating abdominal trauma.Arch.Surg. 133: 1289-1296.

➢ **Tytgat-GN. (1996).** Current indications for Helicobacter pylori eradication therapy. Scnd. J. Gastroenterol. 31 (Suppl. 215): 70-73.

➢ **Tytgat-GNJ. (1994).** Treatments that impact favorably upon the eradication of Helicobacter pylori and ulcer recurrence. Aliment. Pharmacol. Ther. 8 : 359-368.

➢ **Uko-Nne-SD; Mendes-RW; Jambhekar-SS. (1989).** Drug Dev. Ind pharm. 15 (5): 719.

➢ **Umamaheshwari-RB; Jain-S; Bhadra-D; Jain-NK. (2003).** Floating microspheres bearing acetohydroxamic acid for the treatment of Helicobacter pylori. J. Pharm. Pharmaco. 55 (12): 1607-13.

➢ **Umamaheshwari-RB; Jain-S; Jain-NK. (2003).** A new approach in gastroretentitive drug delivery system using cholestyramine. Drug Deliv. 10 (3):151-60.

➢ **Umamaheswari-RB; Jain-S; Tripathi-PK; Agrawal-GP; Jain-NK. (2002).** Floating-bioadhesive microspheres containing acetohydroxamic acid for clearance of Helicobacter pylori.Drug Deliv.9(4):223-31.

➢ **Umezawa-H. (1978).** Pepstatin floating minicapsules, US Patent 4,101, 650.

➢ **Urquhart-J; Theeuwes-F. (1984).**Drug delivery system comprising a reservoir containing a plurality of tiny pills, U.S. Patent, 4.434, 153.

➢ **USP XXIII, (2000).** The United States Pharmacopoeia, NF 18, US. Pharmacopieal Convention, Inc, Rockville, M.D., USA.

➢ **Van Gansheke-B; Timmermans-J; Schoutens-A; Moes-AJ. (1991).**
Intragastric positioning of two concurrently ingested pharmaceutical
matrix dosage forms. Nuel. Med boil. 18: 711-718.

➢ **Walton-BC;Paulson-JE;Argona-MA.(1974).**American   cutaneous
leishmaniasis:inefficiency   of   metronidazole   in
treatment.JAMA.228,1256-1258.

➢ **Warren-SJ; MacRae-RJ; Melia-CD. (1999).** Investigation into the
effect of Weak Acid Modifiers on Improving the Release of
Dipyridanole from Extruded Spheronised Pellets. Proc. Int. Symp.
Control. Rel. Bioact. Mater. 26, 984-985.

➢ **Washington-N; Washington-C; Wilson-CG; Davis-SS. (1986).**
What is 'Liquid Gaviscon'? A composition of four international
formulations, Int. J. Pharm.34: 105-109.

➢ **Watanabe-K; Machida-Y; Takayama-K; Iwata-M; Nagai-T et
al., (1993).** Preparation and evaluation of intragastric floating tablet
having pH independent buoyancy and sustained release property,
Arch. Praet. Pharm. Yakuzaigaku.53: 1-7.

➢ **Weiner-K; Graham-L; Reedy-T; Elashoff-J; Meyer-J. (1981).**
Simultaneous gastric emptying of two solid foods, Gastroenterol. 81 :
257-266,

➢ **Wei-Z; Yu-Z; Bi-D. (2001).** Design and evaluation of a two-layer
floating tablet for gastric retention using cisapride as a model drug.
Drug Dev. Ind. Pharm. 27 (5):469-74.

➢ **Wheeler-LA; DeMeo-M; Halula-M. (1978).**Use of high pressure
liquid chromatography to determine plasma levels of metronidazole
and metabolites after intravenous administration.Antimicrob
.Agents.Chemother.13,205-209.

➤ **Whitehead-L; Collett-JH; Fell-JT. (2000).** Amoxicillin release from a floating dosage form based on alginate. Int. J. Pharm. 210: 45-49.

➤ **Whitehead-L; Fell-JT; Collett-JH; Sharma-HL; Smith-AM. (1998).** Floating dosage forms: an in vivo study demonstrating prolonged gastric retention. J. Control. Rel. 55, 3-22.

➤ **Wibawa-JID; Shaw-PN; Barrett-DA. (2001).** Quantification of metronidazole in small volume biological samples using narrow-bore high performance liquid chromatography. J. Chromatogr. B. Biomed. Sci.25; 761, 213-219.

➤ **Wilson-CG; Washington-N. (1989).** The stomach: its rote in oral, drug delivery, in: M.H. Rubinstein (Ed.) physiological pharmaccuties: Biological to drug absorption. Ellis Horwood, Chichester, pp. 47-76.

➤ **Witehead-L; Fell-JT; Collett-JH. (1996).** Development of a gastro retentive dosage form. Eur. J. pharm . Sci. 4 (Suppl.) S 182.

➤ **Wong-W; Hodge-MG; Lewis-A. (1994).**Resolution of cyclosporin-induced gingival hypertrophy with metronidazole (letter).Lancet.343, 986.

➤ **Wood-BA; Monro-AM. (1975).**Pharmacokinetics of metronidazole and tinidazole in women after single large oral doses.Br.J.Venereo.Dis.51, 51-53.

➤ **Xu-G; Groves-MJ. (2001).** Effect of FITC-dextran molecular weight on its release from floating cetyl alcohol and HPMC tablets. J. Pharm. Pharmacol.; 53(1):49-56.

➤ **Xu-WL; Tu-XD; Lu-ZD. (1991).** Development of gentamicin sulfate sustained-release tablets remaining floating in the stomach, Yao Hsuch Hsuch Pao 26: 541-545.

➢ **Yange-L; Fassihi-R. (1996).** Zero-order release kinetics from a self-correcting floatable asymmetric configuration drug delivery system. J. Pharm. Sci. 85: 170-173.

➢ **Yeung-PKF; Little-R; Jiang-YQ; Buckley-SJ; Pollak-PT; Kapoor-H; Veldhuyzen-Van-Zanten-SJO. (1998).** A simple high performance liquid chromatography assay for simultaneous determination of omeprazole and metronidazole in human plasma and gastric fluid.J.Pharm.Biomed.Anal.17, 1393-1398.

➢ **Yuasa-H; Takashima-Y; Kanaya-Y. (1996).** Studies on the development of intragastric floating and sustained release preparation. I, Application of calcium silicate as a floating carrier. Chem. Pharm. Bull. 44: 1361-1366.

➢ **Zimmerman-J; Silver-J; Shapiro-M. (1988).** Clindamycin unresponsive anaerobic osteomyelitis treated with oral metronidazole .Scand.J.Infect.Dis.12,79-80.

➢ **Zuirbis-P; Socholisty-I; Kondritzer-AA. (1956).** J. Am. Pharm. Ass. Sci.Ed. 45,450.

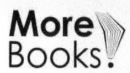
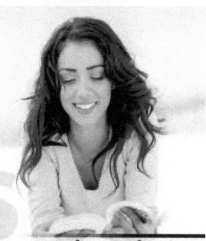 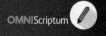

Printed in the USA
CPSIA information can be obtained
at www.ICGtesting.com
LVHW090148140923
758170LV00008B/57